Women's Health Guide

*A Natural Approach to Breast Cancer,
Heart Disease, Fibroids, PMS,
Bulimia, Childbirth, Menopause,
and Osteoporosis*

Edited by Gale Jack
and Wendy Esko

One Peaceful World Press
Becket, Massachusetts

In memory of Lily Kushi

For further information on mail-order sales, wholesale or retail discounts, distribution, translations, and foreign rights, please contact the publisher:

One Peaceful World Press
P.O. Box 10
Leland Road
Becket, MA 01223
U.S.A.

Telephone (413) 623-2322
Fax (413) 623-8827

First Edition: May 1997
10 9 8 7 6 5 4 3 2 1

ISBN 1–882984–25–0
Printed in U.S.A.

Contents

Introduction
by Gale Jack

Rates of degenerative disease are rising more rapidly in women than in men. In the United States, breast cancer incidence recently rose from 1 in 9 women to 1 in 8 in less than two years, and it has been declared an epidemic in many regions. Lung cancer rates, associated with higher fat consumption and smoking, are increasing more rapidly in the female than male population.

Heart disease remains the greatest threat to women's health, killing between one in two and one in three women. Younger women are more immune than men because of menstruation, but by age sixty-five a woman's risk of suffering a heart attack is almost the same as a man's. Moreover, women are twice as likely to die as men after a heart attack and are less likely to survive surgery and other conventional treatments.

Though women live longer than men, they are sick longer. "We appear to be trading longer life for worsening health," explains a researcher at the Argonne National Laboratory. A recent issue of the *Journal of Aging and Health* concluded that because many more people, especially women, are expected to live into their 70's, 80's, and 90's, they are apt to suffer from arthritis and Alzheimer's disease, and the overall health of the population is worsening. On average, according to a study published in the *Journal of Health Psychology*, American men have a life expectancy of 60 years in good health and 12 years in poor health, while women have 63 in good health and 16 in illness.

On the plus side, women are generally more aware of alternative approaches to health than men and are more likely to change their diet and try other holistic therapies.

For the last thirty years, Michio and Aveline Kushi's pioneering work has guided thousands of women, children, and families to greater health and happiness. The macrobiotic way of life that they introduced has now spread throughout modern society and is beginning to find greater acceptance in the medical community as well as among mind/body researchers.

The *Women's Health Guide* is the first book completely devoted to women's health from a macrobiotic perspective. It features a wealth of practical information that the ordinary woman can immediately put into practice as well as inspiring case histories of women around the world who have healed themselves of serious illnesses with the help of a more balanced diet and lifestyle. Articles, essays, and interviews with leading teachers, counselors, and physicians in the field complement the first-person accounts. At the end, there is an appendix summarizing recent scientific and medical research on diet and women's diseases, as well as a resource section, bibliography, and index. The new Women's Health Seminar at the Kushi Institute, described in the resource section, is especially recommended.

Looking back, I wish I had access to this information about twenty years ago when I started macrobiotics. It would have saved me a lot of heartache and pain. Still, I was able to heal myself of ovarian tumors without surgery (as my doctors recommended) and pass through menopause symptom-free. I am endlessly grateful for macrobiotics and hope that this book will benefit you in your journey through the stages of life.

Gale Jack
Becket, Massachusetts
February 7, 1997

Chapter 1
Women's Health Forum

Through a more natural way of life, including a more healthful way of eating, many women have prevented and relieved serious illnesses. This chapter presents the personal accounts of ten women who have observed a macrobiotic diet and lifestyle to heal conditions ranging from cancer and immune deficiency diseases to bulimia, hepatitis, and endometriosis. For further biographical information, please see the Contributors section at the end of this book.

Crohn's Disease and Takayasu Arteritis
by Virginia Harper

"You can turn this around. You can change this," are the words I'll never forget. After eight years of living with Takayasu arteritis and Crohn's disease and seeing only a dim future ahead, these words filled me with hope.

At age fourteen, I started having strong symptoms of discomfort and pain on the right side of my abdomen. At fifteen, they removed my appendix but discovered it was normal. From fifteen to twenty-three, I was in and out of hospitals at least twice a year with the symptoms getting more severe. I had not only the increasing abdominal problems but I started to develop fainting spells, dizziness, weakness in my right shoulder and arm down to my hand. At age nineteen, I discovered a lump on my neck. I was away at college in Tennessee and the school doctor decided it was a benign cyst and could be easily removed during the Thanksgiving holidays.

While undergoing an arteriogram at home in Connecticut, I suffered a stroke. When I awoke, I was temporarily paralyzed on my right side and had lost my ability to speak. The test showed a blockage on my right carotid artery. In April of that next year, I was sent to Massachusetts General Hospital in Boston to undergo bypass surgery and a biopsy and it was determined that I had a very rare blood condition. Takayasu arteritis is an autoimmune deficiency where the blood passing through the arteries causes them to act as if they are damaged so they start repairing themselves and this creates blockages. Takayasu has no known cause and no known cure. The main arteries were so dramatically affected that my blood flow was distressed. I was told to stop all my sports activities and "to take it easy." But the real devastating news was that I should not plan on having children.

I was put on an anti-inflammatory drug called prednisone, a sterol, and an aspirin a day to help with my blood flow. The next few years I learned to live within the confines of Takayasu and I suffered from the side effects from the drugs more than the disease itself. I would awaken ravished with headaches, swollen aching joints, ringing in my ears, upset stomach, low energy and feelings of depression. And, when I was on high doses, I would be so hyper I would work to exhaustion and still only need three or four hours of sleep before I was ready to go again.

On top of all this, my abdominal symptoms began to get worse as the years went by. The pain became paralyzing, along with constant headaches, bloody diarrhea, constipation and weight loss. At times I would lose so much blood that I would go to the emergency room completely debilitated. The X-rays showed nothing. Eight years of different doctors, specialists, tests, and drugs, yet the cause and cure were still a mystery.

Finally, when I was twenty-two, I had a severe attack which landed me back in the emergency room. But this time, the technicians were finally able to detect something on the X-rays. The doctors diagnosed Crohn's disease. I was so relieved to have a name for what I had gone through all those years. Crohn's disease has no known cause and no known cure. It causes a slow deterioration of the intestinal wall, the lining becomes inflamed and irritated, and loses its elasticity, resulting in impaired digestion and absorption. Crohn's can manifest anywhere in the digestive tract.

Anti-inflammatory drugs and/or surgery were the only recourse. Surgery can remove the affected area; however, Crohn's usually spreads again in three years or less and more surgery is necessary. It didn't take me long to realize that if I lived to be thirty, I would not have any intestines left.

The "good news" was that I was already taking the anti-inflammatory drug used to treat it. When I inquired how I could develop something so severe when I was already on the drug that supposedly helped it, I got no response. And so, I learned to live within the confines of Crohn's and prednisone.

To complicate matters, that same year I became pregnant while using the IUD. Instead of this being a happy time for my husband and me, it was quite traumatic. The doctors thought I would lose the baby when they removed the IUD. However, the pregnancy continued and went smoothly while the doctors watched me very closely and I stayed in bed most of the time. Being as determined as I am, our beautiful daughter was born.

Nine months later, the Takayasu and the Crohn's both flared up again and so did my trips back to the hospital and doctors for more tests and different drugs, except this time nothing seemed to work for very long. My parents and I, being open to alternative methods, started searching for real cures. I tried megavitamin therapy, reflexology, herbs, and hospital-based nutritional approaches. It was during this search that my father heard about macrobiotics. He cried as he told me what would work this time and shared what little he knew. He flew me to Connecticut to see a macrobiotic teacher. I was ready to deal with this doctor, too. I took all my X-rays, files, and paperwork to show him, but the experience was totally different.

He wanted to know specific details of my symptoms and my lifestyle. There was no prodding, poking, sticking, undressing, or cold intrusive instruments to deal with. He used

9

Oriental diagnosis to evaluate my condition by observing my eyes, tongue, hands, and feet.

Finally, he told me what I had longed to hear, "You can turn this around." The macrobiotic teacher proceeded to explain that there were certain foods that weakened my body and it was struggling to get rid of excess. All my body needed were the correct tools to naturally heal itself. The main foods that aggravated my condition were dairy food and sugars. For maximum health, he explained the importance of keeping the blood alkaline by eating neutral or balanced foods. These include whole grains, beans, land and sea vegetables, and some fruit, seeds, and nuts.

I grew up with my grandmother and she strongly believed that God's abundance provides everything one needs to naturally heal. All I heard finally was making sense. I did not recognize half of the foods he mentioned because, after all, I was a fast-food, junk-food, pre-prepared, vegetable-come-in-a-can baby boomer.

I had ANSWERS and most of all for the first time, I had hope. My teacher told me that one day I would appreciate and be thankful for my illness. I thought, "This guy has been eating too much seaweed—he just doesn't realize all I've been through!"

Now, 15 years later, I continue to live a symptom-free, drug-free, pain-free, doctor-free life. Full of energy, I anticipate a health-filled future with my two children and family. I truly understand those prophetic words. I do appreciate my illness and all I went through. My experience led me to macrobiotics and that led me to the path of healing physically, emotionally, and spiritually. And that quality of healing you can never get from a pill.

Hepatitis
by Yuko Horio

In August, 1987, when I was thirty-four, I was traveling through South India with my partner, Toru, for two weeks just after the monsoon season. The daytime temperature was around 99 to 100 F. (37-38 C.). It was hot and hard to travel. In Tokyo the temperature was normally around 86 F. (30 C.), even in midsummer.

I already had practiced macrobiotics for seven years, but not strictly. I had eaten some dairy food and refined bread for breakfast and occasionally ordinary food outside because there were few macrobiotic restaurants in Tokyo. Nevertheless, I had confidence in my health, as this was our fourth trip to India, and we often took umeboshi plums during the journey.

Under the red-hot sun, we turned to tropical fruits, chai (hot tea with milk and sugar), and sugar cane juice with ice, which was made by vendors who put sugar cane through a wringer. It tasted like nectar. Needless to say, many flies swarmed around us, but I didn't care, as I believed I would never get sick.

After several days passed, I began to feel quite tired. I lost my appetite and experienced some diarrhea. I craved liquid, and whenever I found a vendor of sugar cane juice, I bought some. I could barely follow Toru on the rest of the trip. I went from 115 pounds to 110.

Even after returning home, I had no appetite, preferred to drink juice, and felt disoriented. This went on for a month. At the end of September, the weather cooled drastically and I got a slight fever. I thought it was a cold.

On October 3, I felt very sick and had no energy. Even looking at food made me nauseated. I vomited milk tea at noon that I had drunk in the morning. The condition persisted. At the hospital, doctors took tests and gave me an I.V. I took medicine for three days to be able to eat brown rice again. I ate rice carefully, chewing 100 times and sangoso

11

powder, or glaswort, which grows by the seaside and is high in minerals. My body seemed to be recovering, but jaundice set in. In a medical book, I read that hepatitis type A is contracted by ingestive infection through food or drinks. I thought about my trip to South Asia. I realized I had hepatitis A and resigned myself to be hospitalized.

As I awaited my test results, Tastunori Murakoshi, a macrobiotic friend, called. I told him my story and he reminded me, "There isn't any illness that cannot be relieved by food." I decided to follow his advice.

My blood tests indicated liver imbalance. It was acute hepatitis. Naturally, the doctor wanted to hospitalize me immediately. When I tried to leave, saying I would discuss it with my family, he said there was no time. When I persisted, he became irritated, ordered a nurse to bring a medical book, and showed me the section that said if my condition changed to fulminant hepatitis I would probably be dead within a week. Also a nurse told me she had never seen such high liver-function levels before. My GOT was 4190 (normal is 8 to 35), and my GPT was 3130 (normal 3 to 30). She had never seen anyone's over 2000. The doctor told me that he would treat me with steroids.

Finally, I managed to leave, and at home started to practice a strict macrobiotic diet. I ate brown rice, gomashio, miso soup with seaweed, cooked konnyaku (dried gourd), some other simple dishes, and sangoso powder and chewed my food more than 100 times. At that time, my urine's color was coffee-like. Kan Tomoi, another macrobiotic friend, came to see me and told me I had to eat humbly and exercise well to improve my metabolism.

Even though my jaundice progressed and my weight decreased, I started to feel better day by day. In the process, I missed my period and experienced painful stomach convulsions for the first time in my life. With Toru's help, I treated them with loquat leaf and boiled konnyaku. I was able to go to the library but didn't go to work.

On October 20, I returned to the hospital. A different doctor greeted me, but his face turned grim when he saw my chart and heard the explanation of my own therapy. "I won't perform your blood test today," he said. "Such an unnutritious diet doesn't work." Finally, he agreed to give me a blood test. The results were: GOT 82; GPT 84; and ALP 1040 (normal is 100 to 280). The urine had returned to a natural color. By the end of October, I returned to work. In the middle of November, I was examined again and the results were almost normal. Later I had a blood test at my company's health check-up, and I tested negative for hepatitis B antigens. This suggested I had type A as I thought.

Incidentally, though one doctor couldn't believe my subsequent blood test levels, I have some evidence, as a kind of sequel, which shows that my story of dietary recovery is true. My ZTT and TTT, also liver-function tests, are a bit higher than normal range even now. The figure, however, is decreasing gradually each time. When I first received the results that showed my liver function was abnormal, I was shocked. But now I find that they are very precious in helping me stay with the macrobiotic way of life.

ITP—Idiopathic Thrombocytopenia Purpura
by Joan Young

As I stood on the top of the expert slope in Colorado, skis pointing downward, breathing in the fresh spring air, my thoughts could not help but drift to how different I felt from last year. In January the prior year I remember lying in the family room watching TV and being envious of the people on the screen. Unlike me, they had hair. They could walk up stairs without being winded or having chest pains. They could do their own cooking and laundry. They could visit friends. They could form coherent thoughts. They were not on medication that dulled their senses and made them a stranger to their friends and family.

My debilitation began in June the year before. I had what I thought was the flu but didn't recover as I usually did. I was constantly fatigued. Then I noticed some bruises that appeared with no injury to that area. I bit my tongue and it didn't stop bleeding for a long time. I brushed my leg against a corner of a table and had a large black and blue mark. I went to a party and ate some pizza and drank some beer and knew that the party food was not helping me. I continued working hoping that I would somehow just recover and the strange happenings would stop.

In an effort to continue to lead a normal life, I went on a long planned business trip to San Francisco hoping the bay air would revive me as it had on past trips. I found myself wanting to escape the basement rooms of the conference and walk in the sun. I searched for vegetables to eat. I was drawn to those shops in Chinatown that displayed strange remedies in the windows and had drawers of herbs. I wanted to go in and ask the venerable Chinese men behind the counters why my body was behaving so differently and could they please fix it. I never had the courage.

I returned, happy to be home, and decided to go to a doctor. The diagnosis was ITP—idiopathic thrombocytopenia purpura. *Idiopathic* meant that there was no defined cause, *thrombocytopenia* meant that I had a low platelet count, and *purpura* meant that there was an appearance of purpura, black and blue marks. It was an autoimmune disease in the same class as lupus, multiple sclerosis, or rheumatoid arthritis. For some reason, my body had decided that my platelets, necessary to form blood clots, were foreign. It formed antibodies and eliminated them. My spontaneous black and blue marks were really spontaneous hemorrhaging. ITP is usually not a fatal disease. However, with extremely low platelet counts, I was susceptible to a spontaneous brain or gastrointestinal tract hemorrhage. The normal platelet range is 150,000 to 400,000. The minimum amount needed to prevent the hemorrhaging is 30,000. My platelet count was 6,000.

The doctor suggested that I go to the hospital immediately for some tests and begin taking prednisone, the drug therapy of choice for this condition. The tests confirmed the diagnosis and I reluctantly consented to take the drug, wary of the listed side effects of diabetes, paranoia, osteoporosis, and seizures.

The drug therapy did not work. My platelets did not rise as expected. As I was weaned off the drug, I had something that was later diagnosed as a potential heart attack, then a seizure. In the hospital, I had a resting pulse of 120. Now in addition to a hematologist, I had a neurologist, a cardiologist, and mounting medical bills. I was taking a heart drug, an anti-convulsant drug, and IVIG, an intravenous therapy for my platelets. My platelets were not much better than when I started the cure.

Each day passed in a blur. Sometimes my breathing was so slow I had to remember to take another breath. At night, when I was falling asleep, my mind seemed to go to some deep dark place unlike anything I remembered before. I was afraid that I would not wake.

The IVIG treatments, while initially beneficial, no longer raised my platelets. I had my spleen removed. This did not have a long term positive effect. I took colchicine and danocrine, other drugs. None of it helped for long, and each treatment took its toll on my body.

As the treatments became less beneficial and there were fewer possibilities, I began to search for alternatives. I had my food allergies checked and eliminated those on the list including tomatoes, dairy, and additives. My platelets seemed to stabilize.

I went to a psychologist to try to help me deal with the depression, cope with my debilitation, and strengthen my communication with my doctors. She asked me if I considered controlling my disease with diet. I said that I thought I was eating well. She suggested I read Elaine Nussbaum's book, *Recovery from Cancer*. I read the book cover to cover in a few days. I wanted to go out and buy fifty pounds of brown rice. I realized there was a whole new meaning to eating healthy.

Macrobiotics seemed to make sense. I didn't have cancer, but like that disease my body had lost its way. I wish I could say that I changed my diet and everything was wonderful. The truth is that I caught what seemed like the flu and my platelets dipped. I had little choice but to go to the hospital for a platelet transfusion and negotiate with the doctors. I did succumb to a pro-sorba column "blood-cleaner" treatment and vincristine, a chemotherapy drug. Meanwhile, my macrobiotic cooking teacher brought food to the hospital. I was quite a sight in the blood treatment room as the nurse assistant fed me some seaweed because my arms were immobile from the blood machine.

This was January, my final hospitalization, and the final straw in my battle with conventional medicine. My hair fell out. I was so weak from the treatments that I could not go up stairs. I decided to take my chances with the disease and alternative treatments because I knew the modern cure was killing me.

I continued on my diet and gradually felt better. My platelets were holding relatively safe and steady. There was one glorious day when I stood in the sunlight and actually felt my disease shrinking.

I finally had the energy and time to visit Elaine Nussbaum and receive some macrobiotic counseling. She said my disease was easy to diagnose. I was very yin, expanding. After all, my blood was escaping from my body. With her help, I further refined my diet and made it more yang.

I went back to work in April. By mid-summer my platelets were in the normal range and I was off all medications. My hematologist said that it was a spontaneous remission. I had some difficulty with these words since I was spending several hours a day cooking, meditating, receiving Reiki treatments, and doing yoga exercises. Later he said that perhaps I was misdiagnosed, despite the fact that three hematologists confirmed the original diagnosis.

My platelets are holding in the normal range and I'm leading a fulfilling life once again. My energy is restored. I now have the peace of mind I sought for so many years. My friends tell me that I am looking younger than before I was ill. I am more sensitive than ever before to my state of being and now have the knowledge and courage to change the way I feel by the foods I eat and balancing the energies surrounding me. I've met wonderful friends. I've renewed my interest in gardening. I feel close to love and life. I think I finally know why I am here.

Breast Cysts
by Marlene Barrera

For several months, I had felt the desire to have my breasts checked for possible cysts or tumors, but not wanting to expose myself to radiation, I was reluctant to undergo a standard mammogram. In January 1995, after returning from a spiritually oriented trip to India, my intuition continued to tell me that I needed a medical checkup.

On this occasion, a local naturopath offered me the opportunity of undergoing a thermogram, a heat sensing technique which detects densities within the body such as tumors and cysts. This process is regarded by many clinicians as superior to the mammogram due to its capacity for detecting growths at very early stages.

The thermogram indicated a cyst in my left breast and two others forming in my right breast. The naturopath who performed the process was particularly concerned with the growth on the left breast, which appeared to be a serious health problem. I am in my late-30's and, like most women my age, worried about cancer. Although he recommended a treatment based on herbal supplements, I decided to investigate other forms of healing. A close friend suggested a local doctor of Oriental medicine who had success treating cancer patients. His confidence and gentleness with me during a telephone interview assured me that he was the right person to help me heal.

On my initial visit to Dr. Takamatsu, he mentioned that I needed to remove all dairy products from my diet. He stood quietly and looked at me squarely in the eyes as if to see if I could or would reconcile this change in my lifestyle. Since I became a vegetarian, most of my protein was derived from dairy products. I was particularly fond of yogurt and cheese. My desire was to heal, and without hesitation I replied, "Yes." Then almost in the same breath, I asked, "What about sugar?" Don't ask me what possessed me to ask that question, especially since at this point I had no notion of macrobiotics. "No, sugar," he replied. On the treatment sheet he provided an explanation of the macrobiotic diet and a strong encouragement to follow this regime to hasten the healing process.

Nature seemed to take me under her wing, for within a few days I discovered *The Cancer Prevention Diet* by Michio Kushi and a local macrobiotic restaurant. Several weeks later, I met Edward Esko, a teacher and counselor at the Kushi Institute in Becket, Mass., who was giving a lecture at this same restaurant and I arranged with him for a private consultation.

There are many factors involved in healing. I decided to approach my healing process holistically, and thus actively involve mind, body, and spirit in the recovery process. Already I had an established background in practicing contemplation and meditation. For several months, I had learned and practiced pranayamas, or yogic breathing exercises, which oxygenate and detoxify the cells in the body. My experience with massage therapy (I'm a certified massage therapist) had exposed me to both physical de-stressing techniques, as well as various energy techniques such as Network Chiropractic, Reiki, and Cranio-Sacro. I continued acupuncture treatments with Dr. Takamatsu. My weak spots were my past diet and lack of exercise, so I began yoga classes and strictly followed Edward Esko's macrobiotic recommendations.

Although I initially lost a great deal of weight, my energy did not appear to suffer. Not once since starting a macrobiotic diet have I been ill with a cold or flu, or any other ailment. Despite my apparent good health, I felt the need to be reassured about the development of the cysts. Four and a half months after seeking alternatives and beginning to eat macrobiotically, I had a mammogram done (as the thermogram machine was not available). The mammogram revealed fibrocystic tissue, but showed no signs of cysts on either breast.

Actually I am very grateful for my cysts because the experience has exposed me to a healthier way of eating and living. The situation impacted me to the core and has resulted in transformations much greater than are visible in a mammogram. I know of no device yet that can measure the progress of the soul. And yet I can tell you confidently, this form of balanced eating has become an integral part of my soul's evolutionary process.

Breast Cancer
by Christine R. Akbar

My twin sister, Kathy, and I were born September 27, 1952, in Easton, Penn., to our parents, Francis and Arlene Riley. Our ancestry was Irish and Pennsylvania Dutch (German), and our food was typical postwar fare: chicken; eggs; lots of dairy, including ice cream, chocolate, and cheese; sugar; cakes; refined flour; and canned or frozen vegetables. We ate no whole grains like brown rice and never heard of sea vegetables.

From an early age, I suffered from overweight and craved sweets my entire life. I tried many diets in order to slim down, and on one, I ate forty-eight eggs in one week! At age thirty, I adopted a lacto-ovo vegetarian diet, choosing not to kill any more animals. It consisted primarily of cheese omelets, pizzas, ice cream, and chocolate. By this time, I was working hard on a Ph.D. in physics and stayed up all night at least twice a week. My weight had ballooned up to 170 pounds.

My background and degrees in mathematics and science, including a master's degree in high-energy physics, had led to employment in the newly emerging computer field. I had worked in the U.S. and Europe as a programmer, analyst, technical writer, and consultant. In the mid-1980s, I became a teaching assistant in the physics department in my fourth graduate school and served as conference coordinator for the Theoretical Advanced Studies Institute (TASI). I had become disillusioned with Western science, because I had never met an advisor whose ideas made real sense to me and in vain searched for something more meaningful.

In July, 1985, I developed what looked like mastitis. In two weeks, about one quarter of my left breast had become hard under the skin, red, hot, swollen, and painful. Penicillin-type drugs had no effect, and neither a mammogram nor ultrasound revealed anything conclusive. On July 22, a surgical biopsy confirmed inflammatory breast cancer.

I undertook extensive computer research on the current

medical literature for this type of breast cancer, one of the most invasive and deadly. All confirmed that practically no woman was alive two years after this diagnosis in spite of mastectomy, chemotherapy, or radiation treatment. My kind but pessimist oncologist told my husband I might have only two to three months to live, even with medical treatment.

The next day, I started chemotherapy treatments once a month for four months. Side effects included loss of hair in three weeks; nausea; early menopause at age thirty-three; heart palpitations; weakness; and extreme loss of white-blood cells. The inflammatory skin improved after a few treatments, but the diffuse mass of the tumor remained.

In September, my sister gave me a book about a Philadelphia physician who had recovered from terminal cancer using a macrobiotic diet. According to macrobiotics, cancer is caused primarily by a long-time imbalance in our diet and way of life. This made complete sense to me. All my life, I realized that my diet was unhealthful, and I somehow knew that I would become deathly ill. I resolved to recover and lead a life totally different from that of my first thirty-three years.

At home, I immediately threw away all the cheese and chocolate in my kitchen and read ever book I could find on macrobiotics. I began to take cooking classes from a local macrobiotic center in Connecticut and studied yin and yang, the complementary opposite energies that make up all things. I discovered my tumor was caused primarily by the dairy food I was eating. Dairy fat and protein tend to accumulate in the milk-producing part of a woman's body. Meanwhile, the large amount of sugar and sweets I was eating caused the cancer to grow rapidly. I carefully avoided all sweets, oils, and excessive fat and protein; all refined flour products; and ate foods recommened in the breast cancer chapter in *The Cancer Prevention Diet* by Michio Kushi with Alex Jack.

The doctors were amazed at how quickly my body responded to the drugs, how well I overcame side effects, and miraculously how the tumor did not spread like wildfire to the lymph nodes. Although I asked the hospital dietitian for a special diet to reduce my great weight, doctors told me that since I was undergoing chemotherapy, I had to maintain my weight. They said I should eat anything I wanted, especially high protein foods, and recommended a high-calorie chocolate drink.

By now I knew that most doctors had no formal training in nutrition and little idea about the relation of diet and cancer. My intution told me that I should continue my macrobiotic way of eating and studies. Fortunately, chemotherapy produced more yang, contracting effects, offsetting my extremely expansive, more yin condition. I took only a modest amount of drugs to control the acute initial symptoms of the inflammation and then stopped.

Focusing my energy on healing, I stopped my graduate studies and spent every day in the kitchen like an ancient alchemist carefully preparing my meals. My family was supportive and loving and helped carry me through the ordeal.

Further research indicated that radiation treatment twice daily for six weeks could help tumors of this type temporarily. I tolerated the radiation well, especially because I balanced it with additional miso soup and sea vegetables. Despite pressure from my oncologist to resume another six months of chemotherapy, I decided I would rather die than bear more torture of the drugs.

On January 28, 1986, I met Michio and Aveline Kushi at a Kushi Institute seminar and had my first consultation. Aveline kindly presented me with an autographed copy of her new book, *Aveline Kushi's Complete Guide to Macrobiotic Cooking* which I treated like my Bible, and Michio told me in his light, amusing way that I would commit suicide if I ate one more piece of chocolate.

He gave me dietary guidelines tailored to my condition, including four special home remedies: 1) a dish of grated daikon and carrot, which seemed to help me lose weight. 2) A sweet vegetable drink made from onion, cabbage, carrots, and squash, which helped control my sweet cravings. 3) A thick sour drink made from umeboshi plum, soy sauce, kuzu, and water, which probably relieved my chronic constipation which often is a root of breast cancer. 4) A plaster to wear at night on the tumor made of hato mugi (pearl barley) and green cabbage, which helped to soften and draw out excess fat and protein.

As my disease was so far advanced, even Michio was cautious, giving me two diets to choose from: one based on diet alone and the other with diet combined with chemotherapy. Although my husband preferred more drugs, he supported my decision to use only food as medicine. He created a "nest" at home where I could cook peacefully, make special remedies, take walks, sing happy songs, and sleep. He also thoughtfully kept away anyone who brought my energy down, including my well meaning, but pushy oncologist.

For the next two months I observed the healing diet that Michio had recommended. Every second of my time was focused on recovery. I never once doubted that I would live. Macrobiotic philosophy enabled me to understand the energy that had caused the tumor to grow and how to create the energy that would make it dissolve. I learned how food transmutes into blood and what we eat becomes our mind, body, and spirit. With each new meal, I felt my blood grow stronger. Like a cleansing solvent, I visualized it penetrating my remaining tumor and dissolve all the heavy dairy fat and protein that had accumulated. As my body cleansed itself, my intuition became sharper. I began to feel the power of the universe, the forces of heaven and earth healing me directly.

At the end of March, 1986, on Good Friday, I awoke at 4:00 a.m. with nearly uncontrollable diarrhea. I had read that the body sometimes discharges excess animal food in strong ways after starting macrobiotics, so I was not so concerned. But the next morning, to my happy surprise, I realized that the remaining soft mass of my breast tumor was suddenly and miraculously gone!

Within two months under Michio Kushi's guidance, my cancer was gone. In the time that modern medicine predicted I would die, a macrobiotic diet had helped save my life.

In the twelve years since, my health and lifestyle have become more balanced. I had never cheated on my "healing" diet. Gradually, I learned to widen my eating to the "standard" diet and kept daily records of my progress. Following studies at the Kushi Institute in Becket, Mass., I served as cocoordinator for the Way to Health Program, a one-week residential seminar designed to help people, primarily cancer patients and their families, begin macrobiotics. Because of my science background, I was often called upon to represent the Kushi Institute at medical gatherings. For the last several years, I have served as an assistant to Michio and Aveline Kushi at their home in Brookline, Mass. My duties have ranged from assisting Michio with consultations to gathering materials for the National Institutes of Health (NIH) study on macrobiotics and cancer.

My life-long interest in science led me to study transmutation, the macrobiotic theory that heavier elements such as iron can be formed from common, lighter ones such as carbon and oxygen. According to modern science, such transmutation cannot take place except through nuclear reactions at high temperatures and pressures. However, recent advances in "cold fusion" have stimulated interest in the field.

Following publication of *The Philosopher's Stone*, Michio Kushi's book on transmutation, we began simple experiments at the Kushi residence, and this year Michio appointed me director of the Kushi Foundation Transmutation and Energy Center. Just as cancer, heart disease, and other illnesses can be healed with peaceful, gentle means, it is our hope that someday unlimited sources of energy and scarce metals will become commonly available and help heal the planet. I am grateful for my family, my teachers, and for the great gifts of long life and the unifying principles of nature given to me by macrobiotics, the way of health, happiness, and peace.

Chronic Fatigue
by Lucy Burdo

Growing up I was always healthy, and my teenage years were filled with soccer, cross country ski racing, dance, gymnastics, and outdoor exercise. When after starting college six years ago, I could barely make it through my daily dance classes without exhaustion, I knew my health had seriously deteriorated. Even with my will to push my body as hard as I could, it took a supreme effort to keep myself from fainting or collapsing on the floor from weakness, dizziness, and a chronic fever and sore throat.

These symptoms had been slowly emerging. While still in high school, I developed swollen lymph glands in my neck which didn't recede no matter how much vitamin C I took. And my bouts of sore throats, fever, and general low energy had been increasing. I had visited a homeopath and a chiropractor with some degree of improvement, but still was steadily declining. But nothing could have prepared me for the total loss of health I experienced in January, 1990.

After a week at college for a new semester, I physically couldn't get up in the morning. I had to drop out of school immediately. I had severe night sweats and a chronic fever. When I was able to get up around 11:00 A.M., I was barely able to cook for myself. I visited my physician who suggested that there was nothing physically wrong with me as I wasn't in a wheelchair. I should accept that I had no energy to function. The only treatment he could suggest was to remove my swollen lymph glands. However, in a later conversation, he suggested that I had chronic fatigue syndrome, and might benefit from alternative medicine.

One of the alternative health care providers I consulted performed "live blood cell analysis" on a drop of fresh blood extracted from my finger. Apparently this is a popular test in Japan and is useful in getting a complete picture of the functioning of the blood and overall health. As we saw the cells come into focus on the video monitor hooked up the microscope, the practitioner turned to me and exclaimed, "I don't know how you're sitting here. You're going on will power alone." My white blood cell count was low, and the cells were poorly formed and were dying almost as soon as they were born. They were so overloaded trying to escort toxins out of the immune system that they would break and spill their load right back into the blood sample we were watching.

Next we examined the red blood cells. They were small and poorly formed also. Furthermore, there were huge clumps of candidias yeast drifting through them. My blood wasn't able to do its job, and my immune system was incredibly weak.

24

I left with images of my weakened T-cells and poorly shaped red blood cells fresh in my mind and armed to the gills with all sorts of symptomatic remedies to boost my immune system and strengthen my blood cells. These included Chinese herbs, shark liver oil, and homeopathic remedies for radiation and environmental toxins. This was to be my inspiration and gave me the visual imagery I needed to heal.

Fortunately, about two weeks earlier, my boyfriend's mother had given us a Christmas/Hannukah gift of a consultation with a macrobiotic counselor. This proved to be the catalyst toward health and my saving grace. As we drove to Massachusetts, my intuition told me this was my chance to get a piece of the big picture. I also knew that if this didn't hold the key, I might never know how to regain my health. Symptomatic cures were no longer effective; I needed to go to the heart of my illness, the roots and causes and address them.

The counselor patiently answered "no" as I asked him if all my favorite foods were included in the daily macrobiotic diet. I learned that no tomato sauce, soy cheese, brewer's yeast, chocolate chip cookies, ice cream, or grilled cheese sandwiches were included. As we were going out the door, I felt my energy fading rapidly and accepted a simple looking fresh rice ball as a snack. Although desperate, I wouldn't usually have settled for a plain snack. A chocolate bar or cookies were what my hands reached for, even as my intuition lodged a quiet protest. Imagine my surprise when I felt my energy come slowly, steadily, and evenly back.

I arrived home filled with curiosity about this new diet and cooked my first macro meal of chickpeas, short grain brown rice with umeboshi paste as a condiment, and boiled broccoli. As I was eating, I felt some energy clear around my head, as if coming out of a dense fog. I wouldn't have paid attention, except that my boyfriend said, "Lucy, this may sound weird, but I just felt all this energy clear around my head as if a fog lifted."

Hello umeboshi! Well, the experience of this meal spoke to something deep inside me, and I realized then and there from the inner recesses of my soul that I was going to be macrobiotic the rest of my life. Since I had the rest of my life, I decided to allow myself to transition slowly and gently. For breakfast and lunch, I enjoyed eating very plain, very boiled macro meals, while for dinner I pulled out all the stops. I was working evenings in a four-star restaurant where I ate widely, including sugary fruit tarts, mocha butter cream cakes, rabbit in cream sauce, and macaroni and cheeses. When I completely crashed three weeks later, I had already begun to transition onto a path and diet which were to be my lifeline, sustaining my body and thus my soul.

I took the approach that healing from this debilitating illness was the most important thing in my life and had to be my total focus. Now that I knew what to do to make myself feel better and regain my health, I would do whatever I had to heal. I didn't have anyone to pay my rent, so practically speaking, my decision was one of necessity. I quit sugar (one of the hardest things I've ever done, but that's a whole other discussion!) and ate boiled rice, tofu, vegetables, and beans for three months. In the beginning, after I'd quit sugar and was experiencing daily the benefits of more energy, I would have intense cravings for cookies, ice cream, or a blueberry muffin. I would make a conscious choice to not eat the sugar, as I so clearly connected the fact that if I did, I wouldn't be able to get out of bed or function the next day. And I treasured having this new energy to get up. Sometimes I would stand there and cry, as I had not yet learned how to cook healthier sweets for myself at home.

After about two months, I remember feeling 20 minutes of real wellness and health coursing through my body and mind! I was out cross-country skiing with two friends, trying to be a good sport as I dragged myself along, unsure if I could go another 20 feet. All of a sudden, a wave of well being hit me, emanating from deep within. I stopped in exclamation and shared my experience, relishing each moment of exhilaration. After all the depression, despair, and monotony of helpless, hopeless feelings engendered by not being able to function physically, this feeling surprised and totally inspired me. I imagined feeling that way all the time! And today I do.

It was an arduous road at first, and the key was macrobiotics. As I got tired of boiled rice, boiled broccoli, and boiled tofu, I took cooking classes and bought cookbooks. The food became new, exciting, and creative. My health improved slowly with many dips and curves along the way.

Since I took the complete approach of including my mental, emotional, and spiritual health, I also visited my chiropractor, therapist, and energetic bodyworker regularly for support. I took responsibility for myself on all these levels and found they all complemented and enhanced the other levels. But the foundation of my new attitude and lifestyle was macrobiotics.

Today I see macrobiotics as a lifestyle which includes all the energy I take in from the environment, not just food. I'm deeply grateful and happy to have been able to create dynamic health in my life through macrobiotics.

Lymphoma
The Kathleen Roeder Story
by Janet Benton

When Kathleen Roeder, R.N., of Aurora, Colorado, went to the doctor in 1981 at the age of forty, she knew something was very wrong. She was suffering from terrible fatigue, her skin was gray-white, and she had dark circles under her eyes. Add night sweats, nausea, and pain in the lymph nodes, and you'll understand why the doctor took a biopsy of an enlarged lymph node.

But a surprising diagnosis came back: the lab had found the sample benign. Nevertheless, Kathleen's condition worsened. Formerly an energetic woman who worked hard as a nurse in an intensive care unit, she could hardly walk or swim due to weak spells. "All I had to do was look in the mirror," she says, "and I knew instinctively that the biopsy was wrong."

In the spring of 1982, she returned to the doctor. Her husband suggested that the biopsy from the previous year be sent to another medical center, and this time the diagnosis was non-Hodgkins lymphoma, Stage 1A. The oncologist told

27

Kathleen that she might live another five years, and suggested that she spend that time doing everything she enjoyed. Born in a seaside resort in England, a three-hour drive from the Scottish border, Kathleen speaks in a lovely English-Scottish lilt, and her voice evinces a strong capacity to enjoy life. But the doctor's advice was impossible to follow, as her condition continued to deteriorate. Several weeks later, a huge tumor appeared in her left groin. On removal, it proved to be a nodular, poorly differentiated lymphoma, Stage 3. Then Kathleen had what was to be her last surgery: a lymph node was taken from her neck to confirm the diagnosis.

Since her condition would not respond well to chemotherapy, Kathleen decided instead to do everything she could to strengthen her immune system. Her sister-in-law sent some books on macrobiotics, and after a preliminary consultation in Boulder, Colorado, Kathleen saw Michio Kushi.

"He was very impressive," she recalls. "He had this spiritual quality. He seems to look right through you, or beyond you. He was calm and reassuring. He laid out the dietary and lifestyle changes, and I followed them." Since she and her husband had been eating a diet which emphasized steak, chicken, dairy, cakes, and other sweets, and included very few vegetables, those changes were no small challenge. Cooking classes helped perfect her practice. Her husband adopted most of the dietary changes as well, with better health.

After three months, Kathleen's energy had improved and her nausea had lessened. By six months, the lumps in her lymph nodes were receding, and by eight months, she couldn't palpate any lumps. The night sweats were gone, she looked better, and she felt more vital. Her oncologist was amazed. "He said, 'Whatever you're doing, keep it up,'" recalls Kathleen. And she did. She maintained the diet, studied piano "to bring myself out of my situation and create joy," and read inspirational poetry, which she says "gave me faith in renewal." "It takes a lot of courage to take responsibility for your own health," admits Kathleen. "But I know I would have been dead by now if I hadn't." Soon Kathleen returned to work part-time at the hospital, and she enjoyed a good life for over a decade.

After many years of recovery, Kathleen began what she calls to "cheat on the diet." "I was eating lots of muffins with maple syrup on them, raw salads from the salad bar, potatoes, French fries," she explains. "Oh, I was really going out, and my husband was getting upset. He sees the correlation completely between food and my condition." By two years later, the straying had taken its toll on her well-being. "I was tired and my color was bad," she says, "and then I felt a lump in the back of my neck and was having weak spells." Her oncologist found no suspicious activity, and her blood work was normal. Kathleen went to see Michio, has reformed her diet, and is recovering her energy again.

"I've got a great belief in this diet," she says. "Of course, I do have my fears; this type of cancer goes throughout the immune and lymphatic systems. But I believe the body knows how to heal itself. Macrobiotics is so simple, such a sensitive approach. It's incredible what it can do. As a registered nurse, I would never have believed it."

Kathleen offers this advice to people with cancer: "Seek out others who have been healed. Read books about people who have been healed. Be motivated and actively seek help. Have hope and don't buy into the pessimism of the medical profession. Read all the literature you can, and don't take no for an answer. You can prolong your life. And you do need to be responsible for your own health. If you need to make radical changes in your lifestyle to promote recovery, don't hesitate. Her healing process has taught her self-acceptance, she says, and "to appreciate the simple things in life, like nature. I wake up each morning, glad to be alive."

In closing, Kathleen quotes from one of her favorite inspirational poems: "Believe within your own true self/ When things look dark for you,/ And in the end you're bound to find/ the sun comes shining through." Given her tremendous courage and her decade and a half of impressive recovery through macrobiotics, it is easy to be convinced that Kathleen Roeder knows what she's talking about.

Uterine Cancer
by Gladys Abeashie

At the end of March, 1989, after several months of noticeable decreasing strength and loss of weight, I was diagnosed in Ghana where I live, as having uterine tumors around the cervical and fallopian areas. Menstrual suppression and infections were the symptoms. I was terrified by this abnormal situation. Therefore, I told the gynecologist that I was psychologically upset and emotionally unstable. So whatever you find, I want you to tell me. He agreed and recognized that I am the kind of person who must know the score in order to feel that I have some kind of control, or at least understanding of the situation. He kept his word.

In view of how the tumor was beginning to block the way from the vulva into the other areas, I was in danger of starving. The aim, therefore, was to remove the tumor surgically, but this was not possible because it was associated with major vital organs in the body. The surgeon/gynecologist and pathologist rerouted the abdominal organs lower and around the tumors to allow me to absorb food. He emphasized that this was not a cure. He indicated softly and gently that I would not survive and also informed my husband that I had only had a few weeks or months to live.

The only Savior was God. The average survival time after diagnosis of uterine cancer is four to six month. So when I came home it was to die.

Until one day my husband and Dr. Ofei brought home a newsletter called *One Peaceful World* reading "Macrobiotics for Personal and Planetary Health." There was much news of health and the means by which one could recover from any form of disease or ill health—how to have good faith and eat food to let it be medicine. It was there that Dr. Ofei told me much about the macrobiotic diet and how he uses it to help his former clients from lots of life failures. My husband and I went to his home office—the Macrobiotic Center of Legon—where he counseled us. There were so many people there including young ones and breast-feeding mothers. We were initially disbelieving but a similar close associate had been helped in a case of profuse bleeding. Our attitude was that it would be better to do something than nothing.

Dr. Ofei recommended a restricted diet tailored to my needs and later, after a couple of months, increased the number of foods I could eat. The diet suited me very well, particularly in giving me strength through brown rice and greens. I found the cereal I had every morning for breakfast sustaining. Eventually eleven months after the operation, I was able once again to rejoin my group and do more exercises.

My physicians and other paramedical were amazed that I have survived for five years and am in good health. This is not what the medical textbooks say. They say that the survival rate for all forms of undetected uterine cancer is 0.8 percent.

I am very much indebted and grateful to Alex Jack, Michio, Dr. Ofei and think that because of the macrobiotic diet, my general health has been so good that my own system organs have managed to prevent any secondary appearing in the bowels. Sometimes members of the village communities ask me how I would eat if I were totally cured tomorrow. My only answer is that Father God who works through One Peaceful World affiliates to Michio, Alex Jack and Dr. Ofei, I would continue to eat macrobiotically because, having learned to cook in this way, I find it delicious as well as health-giving.

Endometriosis
by Dawn Gilmour

When I was seventeen years of age I went to the doctor with pain in my back and sides. I also had extremely painful menstruation which had gone on for several years. A blood test and urine samples were taken, but nothing could be found, and I was put on antibiotics and pain killers. In 1969, I went into the hospital for one month with nephritis. Then, in 1972, after complaining for a number of years about the same pain and having been in the hospital four times for observation, I was told that my condition was probably psychosomatic. My doctors also told me that they would "open me up to keep me quiet," and when they did, they found that I had acute appendicitis and a cyst on the right ovary.

I never did feel right after that operation. I became very weak and continued going into the hospital for investigations (D and C), and was continually on antibiotics.

In 1976 it was discovered that I had endometriosis. I also had ovarian cysts and blocked Fallopian tubes. My surgeon, one of the leading female gynecologists in Scotland, tried to persuade me to have a hysterectomy. I was only twenty-four, and was told that with all of the trouble I had had, "it was just useless baggage." I really had to battle with the surgeon not to have the hysterectomy. During the operation, my tubes were cut and "unblocked," and cysts and tissue from the endometriosis were removed. I was then given heat treatment to speed the healing. Large electric pads were placed on the ovarian region. The pads conducted tremendous heat, and I stopped after four treatments because it was causing blisters on my skin and excessive bleeding.

I then went for a second opinion. The surgeon who I saw was shocked at my condition and could not believe that I was still walking around. I was sent immediately to the hospital for rest and observation. This new doctor said that heat treatment should not be used for my condition as it would accelerate the endometriosis. So in 1977, surgery was performed to remove the left Fallopian tube which had collapsed. Cysts were also removed from the ovaries.

I was then put on hormone treatments so as to suppress all menstruation, as this was believed to be a factor in spreading the endometriosis. One month after this operation, I had a pelvic abscess and was rushed by ambulance to the hospital. They could not operate as it was too dangerous. I was placed in intensive care. I was given blood transfusions, could not urinate, and had tubes everywhere. The doctor did not think I would live. After two weeks the abscess burst and began to drain through the bowel. Little did I know that this would mean I would be running to the toilet up to nine times a day for the next month.

I stayed on the hormones for nine months and then decided to stop taking them. I was having severe headaches and pains in my kidneys, and had gone from 91 to 128 pounds. My heart felt very strained. I had no energy and looked like a walking balloon.

In 1978 I went back into the hospital for an investigation to see how things were going. I really felt no difference. It turned out that everything had accelerated and I was back to square one. The surgeon looked at me and said, "I don't know what to say."

During years of illness I had tried many alternative approaches to healing, including acupuncture, homeopathy, herbs, and faith healing. I had also tried eating a vegetarian diet since 1972. Nothing seemed to make any long term difference. I had also seen psychiatrists and was classified as a manic depressive.

I then met a friend who told me about macrobiotics. I decided to go to London to see Mr. Kushi. I felt I could not do any more damage by trying something else. I was so desperate to get well—to feel human again.

Mr. Kushi gave me certain dietary recommendations which I followed. I felt a difference within four days. Physically, I knew it was going to take a little time to get well, but the change in my mental attitude was so dramatic, so quick, I could hardly believe it. It was an overwhelming transformation for me, and my husband was thrilled with his "new wife."

Nine months later I went back to the Royal Infirmary for another internal examination. No endometriosis was found. My doctor, who had performed my previous surgery, thought that my recovery was unbelievable; he was so happy for me and encouraged me to continue on the macrobiotic diet as that seemed to be the thing that was changing my condition.

My last checkup was in September of 1981, just before I moved to Boston. I had an internal examination and Pap smear. Again, the results showed no problems.

I am so grateful to Mr. Kushi, to my husband, who supported me continuously, and to all my friends for their support. Without their compassion and encouragement things would have been so difficult. We must have this support, faith, and determination, and must realize that we are responsible for our own health and that we have the ability to change everything,

Bulimia
by Janet Karovitch

I am thirty-three years old and live in Montreal. Until six months ago, I was bulimic. For five years I had been starving myself all day and binging at night. With each meal, I took enzyme pills to help myself digest, and an abundance of supplements to replace minerals and vitamins I thought I was not getting. After each meal, feeling overfed, I would take two to three laxatives washed down with senna tea laced with psyllium husk powder. My diet consisted of rice cakes, air popped corn, margarine (diet of course), and a variety of nutrasweet products. Spinach and a teaspoon of beans a week helped to ease my conscience.

Progressively my health deteriorated. My hips were almost completely locked in place and my back and left arm were also starting to painfully spasm into very restrictive positions.

I was depressed. I could hardly walk. Every attempt to seek help never got past a 30-second phone call to obscure eating disorder clinics. I would be put on hold after which I'd hang up. I feared being force fed. My will to live was rapidly slipping away.

At this point I was on disability benefits as my work requires being on my feet. Physiotherapy twice a week plus doctors appointments were the only reasons for leaving my apartment.

I was falling apart at the seams. No one could help because no one knew. Living alone helped to conceal my secret. The mask I wore to hide my depression fooled almost everyone, and those who glimpsed the truth kept their distance.

A girlfriend had given me a book, *A Return to Love,* by Marianne Williamson, and I was reading it for the second time when, one afternoon while resting, my heart started to beat out of control. I was able to breathe, but the rapid pounding was resounding loudly in my ears. I felt some pain in my chest and much fear. I breathed myself down to a state of calm and the attack passed. Then everything I read about came into practice. I was on my knees pleading to a divine force I believed in but had never spoken to. I knew I was dying but more than that I knew how much I wanted to live.

Within minutes the answer came. I had a serious problem. I had to confess—to myself and others. After years of twisted appetite patterns, mental and physical breakdowns, I was ready to take responsibility for my own life.

The next morning, I had a difficult, tearful, but soothing conversation with my mother. I promised myself I would make an appointment with my general practitioner the first thing on Monday. In the meantime, I knew Teva was where I had to go.

I had shopped at this particular natural foods store in the past, but this time it wasn't pills I needed. It was help. I was greeted by Guy Lalumiere, a former student and teacher at the Kushi Institute who is a native of Quebec and now working at Teva. He suggested that I cut out certain foods and try others. He wrote down a recipe for Carrot-Daikon Drink and suggested I take it immediately. I also decided to stop taking birth control pills because I had been experiencing bleeding accompanied by painful menstrual cramps for some time. Guy promised to keep in touch and he did.

I eventually learned that I had a weak digestive system (probably from birth). Having been raised on meat, dairy products, and other modern foods, I had difficulty with assimilation and digestion. I never associated lack of energy or lack of self-confidence with my way of eating. However, over the years the symptoms intensified: dizzy spells, exhaustion, mood swings, and overall numbness became more and more frequent. Even after numerous surgeries for the removal of ovarian cysts and kidney stones and the discovery of stomach ulcers, I never attributed any of my problems to my diet or birth control pills—until now.

My eating habits were never a priority. They were an obsession. Work always came first, and my microwave was my best friend. In my mid-twenties, I decided to begin a vegan diet. I felt much better in the beginning, but due to lack of research and balance, I failed. I fell deeper and deeper into physical and emotional anguish.

By the time I met Guy I could hardly eat at all. Semistarvation and binging-purging were the only ways I knew to keep going. I had damaged my intestines so badly over the years I was apparently a hair's breadth away from cancer.

Along with cooking, I have been introduced to Shiatsu massage, ginger compresses, simple exercises, and home remedies. They have also helped me restore my health. My misconstrued image of my body has also shifted. What I once perceived as my overweight body has drastically changed. Now that the bloating and heaviness has subsided, due to carrying undigested food and eating an imbalanced diet, I no longer feel trapped in a body that never felt like my own. Due to all these methods, shared with love and patience, I have almost fully recovered.

Chapter 2
Macrobiotics, Preventive Medicine, and Women's Health
An Interview with Martha Cottrell, M.D.
by Bob Ligon

Dr. Martha Cottrell travels extensively lecturing on health promotion and disease prevention. She was director of student health at the Fashion Institute of Technology in New York for sixteen years and served as the clinical administrator and medical consultant for an AIDS research project in conjunction with the Boston University School of Medicine and the Kushi Foundation. That research project studied the effects of macrobiotics as an alternative and adjunctive therapy for AIDS. She is co-author, with Michio Kushi, of AIDS, Macrobiotics, and Natural Immunity *(Japan Publications, 1990) and contributed to* Doctors Look at Macrobiotics *(Japan Publications, 1988). Dr. Cottrell has recently retired from her medical practice. This article is reprinted from* Macrobiotics Today, *March/April, 1992, used by permission of the George Ohsawa Macrobiotic Foundation, P.O. Box 426, Oroville, CA 95965.*

BL: I thought that we might explore several areas. One is women's issues in health. Another is your background and evolution from a medical doctor to a preventive medicine/ macrobiotic practitioner. And another is your method and style of treatment as a health care practitioner, plus anything else you would like to share.

MC: That covers a lot of ground. Well, my focus at this time in my life is really coming together with women's issues. Nature, in its infinite wisdom, requires the higher order species have a long period of nurturing from infancy to maturity. The female does most of this nurturing. The whole structure in both the animal kingdom and particularly in our human species acknowledges the fact that the female needs to be protected as well as the young so that nurturing can take place until the next generation can get along on its own. The male goes out and fights the wars, hunts, does whatever. But it's the female that has the long gestational period and also has the long period for nurturing and development of the human species.

What I see happening in our society which concerns me so much is that women are so ill. We are seeing epidemic forms of disease among our women that have not been so prevalent before. Now we see the young women getting a lot of the diseases of men—heart disease, strokes, and lung cancer. The cancers are just eating our young women up. We're seeing younger and younger women having hysterectomies from cancer.

BL: Do you have a feeling about what the cause might be?

MC: Well, whatever the cause, I think that what I'm concerned about, first of all, is that there is not an awareness of the importance of this message. We're always talking about diseases and what is the cause of the disease and what is the cure. But we're not looking at the graver and larger picture, which is the deterioration of our health and destruction of our society.

What I'm seeing, from a wholistic perspective, is that we, as women, have left a place in society that was not working really, and now with the women's movement, we've come to a place where we have many more options for self-realization. In the process, we have been literally denying, rejecting, and destroying our reproductive systems, which is almost self-hatred of ourselves as women, in an attempt to be male-like. In so doing, we are destroying the opportunity for continuation of the species.

Traditionally, the female has been the one that has received fertilization, given birth, and nurtured the next generation. And now we see that we are allowing this to happen in the test tube. We are giving over this power that is female to technology. I see more and more infertility, more and more spontaneous abortions, and more early abortions. It seems that we are losing our identity as women. What are we? What is this female energy? What is the power that we have been endowed with? We are losing that power. I'm concerned with that.

BL: How do you see that expressed in the patients that you see? When they have physical conditions, do they also have emotional and psychological concerns?

MC: There is always an emotional overlay with illness. We tend to think we can separate mind, body, spirit, and emotions. But we can't. Anytime there is an illness, I think we have to be very sensitive. As health practitioners, we have to understand the metaphor of their illness, the language of the illness, in order for them to heal. Just addressing the nutritional or stress factors is not enough. We must also come to an understanding of how our emotions have helped to create a particular disease. What does this message [disease] mean? Why does one person develop breast cancer, another cervical cancer, or ovarian cancer, or colon cancer"

To facilitate healing in other people, first of all, we as healers have to be aware of what it is to be healthy ourselves. If we are not attaining that awareness, it's pretty hard to be aware of what's going on in somebody else.

What I see is that the form of the illness can tell us, and the individual, a lot about the areas that need to be worked upon. Breast cancer is an example. I can't think of any woman that has come to see me with breast cancer who, after working with me, has not been able to acknowledge that they've never known how to nurture themselves.

　BL: Why do people come to see you in particular?

MC: Well, you have to realize that by virtue of who I am, I'm going to attract certain kinds of patients. Just the fact that I have a medical degree behind my name, provides people entrée to me. Many, many people come to me with physical problems because it's their entrée. But also, at some level of their consciousness, they have chosen to come to me because they know that I'm operating on a level other than the physical. So whether they are conscious of it or not, they've chosen to come to me because they are available to look at the emotional and spiritual side, the wholistic. They have an awareness that many patients, who just get into the medical model and never get out, don't have.

My practice is very exciting and very stimulating. Most of the time it's extremely rewarding because I can work with patients on many levels—on the physical, the spiritual, the nutritional, the environmental. Even if it's not right at the surface, I just have to dig a little bit and soon I'm hitting pay dirt. If they're really available, we can do some incredible things together.

BL: Could you describe your method of treatment? What is it that you do in your practice?

MC: I mostly facilitate. I don't treat anybody. I help them to get in touch with their own questions and answers. Then I share my opinions and make some recommendations. It's a partnership; we work it out together. So it's a real facilitating, sharing, exploration. I used to treat people before—write prescriptions and things like that.

I don't do that kind of medicine any more. In the past few years I've moved further and further from crisis intervention. Most of what I do in my practice is to facilitate the person in their search for the modality that's most appropriate for their healing. What I'm available to do is to help them find their own answers. I ask patients to bring as much information as they can: their blood work, any kinds of reports, and I ask them to write out their health history. I tell them to bring any concerns or questions and we'll look at all this together. Then I will help them to find their own answers. So it's a type of counseling. And it can vary from doing macrobiotic counseling, to helping them decide whether they want to do chemotherapy or radiation therapy—or, if they are going to have surgery, what they are willing to accept or not accept. It's a real exciting process, exploring options and encouraging them to use their own intuition to determine what the best choice would be for them at that particular time.

BL: What led to your transition? I assume that previously you were considered a mainstream physician who prescribed drugs and surgery.

MC: Yes, I was in a sense, but I've never really been mainstream anything. Even as a little child I questioned. My home was such that my parents encouraged me to question, encouraged me never to be mainstream. I was always brought up to be very suspicious of the way the majority was going. And to always ask myself, "Is this the right direction to go?"

I had a lot of experience before I even went to college. I had two children before I went to college. I had been married for quite a while. I had worked. I had been in life, I had lived life. I didn't go from high school to college to medical school. I went from high school to marriage to being a mother. I experienced my parents' illnesses, my children's illnesses, and my own illnesses. So, in medical school, I was much more mature in many ways than the other students. So just to sit there as a student and swallow anything hook, line, and sinker—that was not where it was at. And that made it difficult for me at times. The whole medical model is to have things poured down your mouth and then you regurgitate it. I wanted to know why. And I was taught that in science you don't ask why, you ask how. And if you ask how, you can manipulate it. I wanted to know why. I wanted to know the cause. So, in spite of the fact that I was always told I couldn't ask why, I continued to ask why.

BL: What was your practice of medicine like when you first started?

MC: I was a family physician. I delivered babies. I was first assistant at all my major surgeries whether it was brain surgery or orthopedics. I did my own minor surgery. And it was a wonderful experience. I kept up with all the postgraduate stuff. I went to conferences. I prided myself on keeping up on what was going on in medicine, always in the first wave. But even at that, I began to observe that no matter what I did, people kept coming back; they didn't seem to get better. They would get one set of symptoms out of the way and they'd come back with another one. Or I would put them on medication that would work and then they would have side effects and I would have to put them on something for the side effects. And I thought, "This is not what I thought I was going to be like in medicine. I thought we were actually going to heal people. And they don't seem to be healing. As a matter of fact, they seem to be getting worse. Now why is that?"

And, even way back in the sixties, for example, I began to notice that women who would come in with vaginal problems would say to me as they were leaving, "I'm not supposed to have sex with my husband, am I, as long as I'm on this medicine?" And I thought, "That's interesting." And I would say, "Well, yes, you're right." I picked up that that was a way of saying, "I don't want to have sex with my husband. Could you give me permission not to?" So I put it in the back of my mind that the next trip around I would have to talk about this with them. I began to ask myself, "What's going on here?"

The next time that patient would come in, I would say, "How are things at home?" What's going on? Is something going on between you and Frank?" And the answer would be, "He's having an affair."

I began to see that there's some connection. So I began to integrate more and more. Teenagers, unmanageable at home, would be brought in and I would say, "What's going on at home and what's going on at school?" And a lot of times, after taking a while, the mother would say, "Well, you know my mother's living with us and I love my mother but she's such a cantankerous old woman and she just butts into the kid's business. And I can't seem to get her to realize that they're not children anymore. She can't tell them you can't do this or that." And I began to see, mmm, the problem there is related.

And patients would come in and say, "You know, Dr. Cottrell, I read this article in *Prevention* or I read this article in *Ms.*, or somebody told me about this, and I'd like to know what you think about it." So I'd say, "Well, let me read it and I'll get back to you." So I would read it. And I became aware that there was a whole body of knowledge out there that I didn't know anything about. And I would say things like,

"Well, I can't see how this could hurt you and if it seems to be helping you, why not?" So I never made them feel like they were idiots or anything like that. I tried to give them my honest opinion. Sometimes I would say to them, "I really think this is a racket. I think you're being exploited. It's up to you, but for myself this doesn't seem legitimate to me." We'd have that kind of exchange.

So then in my own evolution, when my own illness came about because of my lifestyle—and that's a whole other story that I'm going to write one of these days—but when the time came for me to reflect on my own illness and what I was going to do about it, I realized that I didn't want what I had to offer. My patients had made me aware that there were other ways of doing things. So I began to search for alternatives. And it just so happened (you know it's never an accident—when the student is ready, the teacher appears) that I met a bright, young, family doctor right out of residency in Seattle, Washington who was very wholistically oriented. He invited me to go to a conference out in Wisconsin of the American Wholistic Health Association. I had never heard of it. I was scheduled to go to Washington to a regular medical A.M.A.-promoted thing. I said, "Oh, John, I would love to go but I am already supposed to go down here." And he said, "I really think it would be very beneficial if you would go." I had so much respect for him, there was just some energy there that I said OK. I canceled the other one and I went with him. And that really turned my life around. I became aware of a lot of options and it was really fascinating for me.

That was when I began to explore other options. Other people came into my life "accidentally" that told me about this one or that one. And through meeting a female sailor who had a lot of problems with arthritis, a very angry woman, I learned about a lady, Ilana Rubenfeld, who had been doing some work with Feldenkreis, Fitzpearl, and Alexander. I put that in the back of my mind, but I didn't do anything about it. Then when I had my episode of acute inflammatory arthritis and became very ill, Ilana's name came back to me. So I decided I would go find this woman.

My level of consciousness was not very high at that time.

When I went to see Ilana, I said, "I've heard about your work and I'd really like to study with you. I'd like to learn your techniques so that I could help my patients." That was my access point. I could not walk in and say, "Ilana, I need help." It's so interesting how we find our way. So I said, "May I study with you." I want to learn your technique. I want to be a better doctor." She said, "I don't know if I can teach you how to be a better doctor or how to take care of your patients, but I can teach you how to take better care of yourself." That went right over my head. I said, "Well, then are you saying that I can study with you?" I never got off my focus, see. And she smiled and said, "Of course." And I began to study with her. It took me about two years before I got the message that I was there to help myself.

She facilitated the raising of my consciousness and I realized that I need to get out of New York City. I wanted to get to a more natural environment. I was down at the college [Fashion Institute of Technology] compulsively going through the mail and I threw out this little professional journal. Then I quickly grabbed it out out of the trash can for fear I might miss something. I went through it and saw an advertisement for a position in a rural health initiative. So I took it home and I looked at where it was on the map and it looked like a fascinating area.

I went down to Hyde County which is in North Carolina right on the coast, a very rural area. I was there for a year, but in the process, my arthritis flared up and I went to see an orthopedist because I was having so much bursitis in my left shoulder. I'll never forget it, it was excruciatingly painful. I had gone in actually to get an injection because I had had injections of cortisone before. I didn't want to, but it was so painful that I just forced myself to go. I felt I had no alternative. I had to get some help.

While I was sitting in the waiting room, I picked up *The Saturday Evening Post* and read Sattilaro's article. So my shoulder got me to the orthopedist waiting room where I read about him, and I thought, "This is fascinating." And from that began my search for information on macrobiotics.

I finally got hold of some information. At that time I

didn't know how to do anything but boil rice and steam vegetables, which was very boring, but I started getting better. So then I went back to New York. I realized that everything I was doing in North Carolina was acute crisis intervention. I would try to teach people and they didn't want to hear what I had to say. "OK, Doc, that sounds real good, but what can you do for me now?" Can you give me something for this pain. That sounds real interesting, Doc, but you know I've really got to have something for this." And I realized those patients weren't ready for what I had to offer.

So I went back to the college in New York and continued in the administration. I applied and got a year's fellowship in preventive medicine at Mt. Sinai School of Medicine. I continued to study with Ilana Rubenfeld. I searched out and got into the macrobiotic community in New York, through which Michio Kushi heard about me and approached me in 1983 about working with him with the AIDS group. At that point, I began to go to Boston on a regular basis to study with Michio. And I would sit in with the senior counselors when they came to New York. That's how I learned. That's how I taught myself. It's just been an ongoing study since then.

BL: What convinced you that macrobiotic principles might be effective?

MC: What convinced me, like a lot of people, was that here was a fellow medical doctor, Anthony Sattilaro, who had some positive experience with macrobiotics and felt it contributed to his healing process. If this doctor says there must be something to it, I want to look into it. Pure and simple. Sattilaro. Simply because of the little M.D. behind his name, macrobiotics has touched many Western minds.

After that, when I began to read more about macrobiotics, I found it fascinating. Much of what I read, with my Western medical background, made sense to me. The first thing that clicked for me was when I read about the connection of the ears to the kidney. I was taught the same thing in medical school. When you have a deformity of the ear or the ear is sitting in a certain place on the skull, you better be highly suspicious that there's a deformity of the kidney because they form at the same time. So I said to myself, "If this is true, if they knew this 6000 years ago, I want to know what else they knew 6000 years ago that we don't know now." So that's what intrigued me.

As I studied macrobiotics, I would research what was available in Western medicine that might support or disprove macrobiotic ideas. As I went on in my own research in the medical literature and studying macrobiotics, I was excited and amazed at how well they dovetailed, how supportive they were of each other. They're not contradictory, counter to what many people in medicine think.

BL: Then there is a lot of existing documentation in the medical literature to support macrobiotic claims?

MC: Oh, most of what I use in my lectures comes from Western medical research. I just integrated it with macrobiotic thought. That's what's so exciting for me. I felt confused the first few years when I was in transition. I stopped practicing medicine altogether because I could no longer do what I knew how to do. It was like, "I don't want to do what I know how to do, and I don't know how to do what I want to do." So I quit. For three years I didn't practice medicine.

I was very fortunate. Again, things don't just happen, they're always meant to be, in my opinion. At that time at the college we were experiencing tremendous growth. We had to expand rapidly to keep up with the growth of the college. At that time, I was the only doctor. I had one nurse. So I sat down and presented to the administration my needs in order to keep up with the growth of the college. I needed to do more administrative work so I took on more responsibility as the director. I hired a doctor and nurse practitioners and I put them in to do what they were comfortable doing. I did the administration, took my fellowship and learned more about preventive medicine, and then came back to the college and developed a program in prevention and health promotion for the students, staff, and faculty. You see, I was able to manipulate my workplace so that it was balanced for me. I was giving the students the Western medicine they needed, but I couldn't deal with it so I provided somebody that could. And on the other hand, being the director, I had the opportunity to develop a program in health promotion. So that satisfied me.

That was the beginning of my learning how to balance and to integrate and to take care of other people's needs as well as my own. So that's been the journey.

BL: You've talked about prevention and educating children in your lectures. Could you describe your ideas about these areas?

MC: Well, as far as my interest at this time of my life, it's really in women's issues and children's issues. As I said, I feel that if we women can't heal and be healthy, we can't nurture our children and our society, which is the future. And so I'm very committed to supporting women in finding that healthy place. And in some instances this means not having children. In other instances it means trying to be both the chairman of the board and a mother. How can we facilitate that so that a woman can take care of both her needs and the child's needs and the family needs. How can we support our young people in that way? It's just, as I see it, another direction of the extended family. The extended family has to be the workplace and school and society. In a way, its very exciting in that the extended family is going to have to be really extended if we're going to have a healthy society. It's not just going to be blood kin. We have to become universally each other's family.

This is a challenge. What we need to do is to look at the old patterns and update them. The same needs are there and the same solutions are there. They're decked out in a different form, but the principles are there.

And then there are other women who want to stay home and be housewives and mothers and care for their children. We should provide them the opportunity to do that as long as they want to. Politically, I think we have to redirect our economic resources toward providing either tax benefits or economic incentives to help replace a care giver's earning ability, because that person is earning money. That person is putting a great deal into the society. Therefore, society should pay their social security and pay their retirement and pay them a salary for staying home to care for the next generation. The care they give means that we will not have money going for crime, dropouts from school, or emotionally ill people that become homeless and a care on the society. So we have to really value those women who want to stay home and give them the economic rewards they are due.

The way that women were treated in the past and even since the Second World War is that if you didn't work in the workplace, you didn't have any income, then you weren't known to the government. You had no social security. If your husband died, you had no skills, and you were lost. That's not going to work anymore. That will not work.

On the other hand, if our women go to work and our children are being bounced around the way they're bounced around, the children develop different kinds of problems—emotional problems. They're socially handicapped. They lack communication skills and the ability to commit. They fear and distrust one another and they are filled with paranoia, frustration, and anger which manifests itself in destructive behavior and violence. It shows up as self-destructive behavior as well as drug abuse.

So we really do have to realize that providing nurturing environments is part of what we call prevention just as much as providing a health care clinic. Part of a national health program is to see that healthy homes produce healthy citizens who are productive and contribute to the economic health.

It's a real long-term vision of investing in women and children. Otherwise, we're going to end up with an increasingly heavy social debt that we can't possibly keep up with. A premature baby costs something like $8000 or $10,000 a day to keep in a neonatal clinic. Even after that, 70 percent are severely handicapped and severely deformed. We're going to have to provide custodial care for these people. With the medicine and technology we have to keep people alive, they may live 40 or 50 years. We can't afford that. We have to go back to the beginning and provide supportive and nurturing environments, beginning in school—we have to start there because there is no home.

We hear very conservative people talking about nurturing being the responsibility of the home—what home? Our society basically is a conglomerate of dysfunctional families. High divorce rate, child abuse, latchkey kids. What home? The parents come home, they're so tired they can't even cook a meal, much less sit down and listen and know what's going on with their children.

We have to reevaluate the role of the school. The school has to be part of the extended family so that we can teach communications skills beginning from kindergarten or pre-school. We can teach children to negotiate instead of fight. We can teach them to share. We can teach noncompetitive games so that everybody wins. Win-win situations. That has to begin very early because we know from recent studies that children who experience disruptive episodes before the age of three are at great risk of psychosis. Children who experience marked disruptive experiences before the age of six are at very great risk for neurosis. So we have to work with children during the first six years before they even go to school. Day-care has to be more than babysitting; it has to be a positive and stimulating experience.

We are in a most exciting time. We have a lot of examples of what doesn't work and we also have some examples of what can work. We have the incredible opportunity of taking all of this knowledge and doing something really great with it. But, I think things will get worse before they get better. The bigger the front, the bigger the back. If we learn from all of this, I think we have a tremendous opportunity and can come into a golden age of humankind.

Chapter 3
Fibroids and Reproductive Health
by Michio Kushi

This article is adapted from Macrobiotic Pregnancy and Care of
the Newborn, *Japan Publications, 1984. For further information
on the use of macrobiotic remedies, see* Basic Home Remedies *by
Michio Kushi, One Peaceful World Press.*

Fibroids are fleshy growths within or on the wall of the uterus. They consist of masses of fibrous tissue and may be single
or multiple, large or small. They often resemble a group of
marbles.

Fibroids are widespread among women and result from
an extreme diet, especially the overconsumption of foods containing heavy saturated fat such as eggs, meat, dairy products, and poultry, in combination with extremely yin foods
such as sugar, tropical fruits, oil, soft drinks, and refined flour
products. When these items are eaten regularly, mucus and
fat begin to deposit in the body, initially in areas connected to
the outside, such as the sinuses, breasts, lungs, intestines, kidneys, and reproductive organs.

The excess factors in the blood and lymph streams often
solidify into cysts and tumors. When solidification occurs in
the muscle of the uterus, the result is fibroid tumors. Fibroids
often begin as small seedlings. Whether or not they enlarge
depends on the quality and volume of excess that is deposited
in the uterine region. Frequently, they continue growing as
the result of an improper diet and begin to bulge either

through the outer lining of the uterus or through the endometrium. In some cases, they bulge so far that they are pushed out on a stalk.

Fibroids may or may not produce noticeable symptoms. The most common age for symptoms to occur is between thirty-five and forty-five, although women of all ages can experience them. A common symptom is bleeding, especially in the form of heavy or prolonged periods. This happens because fibroids frequently distort the uterus so that the surface area of the endometrium is increased. A greater amount of endometrial lining is produced each month, thereby increasing the menstrual flow. In this case it is also more difficult for bleeding to stop since the normal spiral musculature of the uterine wall is distorted and cannot contract around the blood vessel. Fibroids may grow to become quite large, even to the size of football, and may begin to cause pain as a result of pressing on organs such as the bladder or rectum.

Excessive fat and protein can also accumulate in and around the ovaries, as well as in the Fallopian tubes. There are literally dozens of varieties of ovarian growths, and each is the result of a different combination of excessive factors in the woman's diet. The most common ovarian cyst is the simple cyst which develops when the ovarian follicle does not rupture and release its egg but instead continues growing. These cysts are generally more yin or expansive, and frequently result from the repeated consumption of milk, butter, and other light dairy products, sugar, animal fats, bananas and other tropical fruits, and oily and greasy foods such as pizza.

Another common type of ovarian growth is the dermoid cyst. Dermoid cysts are frequently found in younger women and often contain hair, fatty material, and sometimes hard calcified "teeth." Dermoid cysts are more yang or contracted, and arise primarily from the repeated consumption of foods high in saturated fat, protein, and cholesterol, including eggs, meat, poultry, and cheese. Interestingly, in traditional Oriental medicine, it was believed that eggs were especially harmful to the ovaries.

Dietary Recommendations

In order to dissolve fibroids and cysts, it is important to avoid the extreme foods that cause them to develop. The standard macrobiotic diet, therefore, can serve as the basis for recovery. (Refer to *Standard Macrobiotic Diet* by Michio Kushi, One Peaceful World Press, for a complete description.) Brown rice, barley, millet, whole corn, and other whole cereal grains can serve as the basis of the daily diet. It is better to minimize the intake of hard baked flour products, as these can cause tightness in the body, even if whole grain flours are used. It is also advisable to limit the use of oil to several times per week. A small amount of high quality sesame or corn oil can be used occasionally in cooking.

Among vegetables, leafy greens help dissolve fibroids and can be eaten on a daily or regular basis. Especially helpful are the green tops of edible root vegetables such as daikon, turnip, carrot, and dandelion. Dried shredded daikon is also helpful in melting hard fat deposits and can be cooked several times per week with vegetables such as onion or carrot. In general, it is better to limit the intake of raw salad to occasional use, and to use quickly boiled or blanched salad on a regular basis. Among beans, it is better to use azuki, chickpeas, lentils, and black soybeans, and use other varieties on occasion. Fresh and dried tofu can be eaten regularly, and tempeh can be included several times a week. Bean proteins contain no cholesterol and are preferable to such high-cholesterol foods as eggs, cheese, and meat.

Sea vegetables contain minerals that help the body discharge toxins. Besides using a small volume of sea vegetable such as kombu and wakame in soups or with beans or vegetables, they can be eaten in small side dishes once or twice a week. Arame and hiziki are especially good for this purpose. Nori flakes and other sea vegetable condiments can also be included in the diet.

During the healing process, it is better to limit the use of fruit to a small volume of temperate (not tropical) fruit several times per week if craved. Fruits can be eaten cooked, dried, or when craved, fresh in season. The intake of fruit juice is best kept moderate. Vegetable such as squash, cabbage, onion, daikon, carrot, parsnip, and others with a naturally sweet flavor can be eaten regularly to ease the craving for sweets. Dried chestnuts are available at natural food stores and when cooked with brown rice or in purées have a delightfully sweet flavor. They can be enjoyed several times per week, together with a small volume of such natural sweeteners as rice syrup, barley malt, and amasake (sweet rice milk.)

Nuts and nut butters, which contain plenty of oil and fat, are best avoided during the first month of so, as are all animal foods. Low-fat white meat fish is the exception, and can be eaten once every week or ten days if craved.

Daikon Hip Bath

Together with a balanced natural diet, the daikon hip bath is a very effective remedy for fibroids, cysts, and other female reproductive disorders. It helps melt stagnation and dissolve protein and fat accumulations in the pelvic region and lower body as a whole. In addition to fibroids, it can be used to help endomitriosis, blocked Fallopian tubes, yeast and bacterial infections, vaginal discharges, and cervical dysplasia.

Ideally, the bath water should contain dried leafy vegetables such as daikon or turnip greens. Dried daikon leaves are available from macrobiotic mail order companies, or you can prepare your own. To prepare, remove the green tops from fresh daikon and hang up in a pantry or other room in your house so that they are not in direct sunlight. Leave them until they turn brown and brittle. If you cannot locate daikon or turnip greens, you may substitute arame sea vegetable.

Place about four to five bunches of dried leaves or a double handful of arame in a large pot. Add about four to five quarts of water and bring to a boil. Reduce the flame to medium and boil until the water turns brown. Add a handful of sea salt and stir well to dissolve.

Then, run hot water in the bathtub and add the mixture together with another handful of sea salt. (You may strain the mixture through a strainer.) Add only enough water to cover your body from the waist down. Sit in the tub and cover your upper body with a thick cotton towel to prevent chills and absorb perspiration. If the water begins to cool, add more hot water and stay in the bath for about fifteen minutes.

The hot bath will cause your lower body to become very red as a result of an increase in circulation. This along with the heat and minerals in the water will loosen fat and mucus deposits in the lower body.

After you finish with the bath, you can prepare a special douching solution. The douche helps dislodge deposits of mucus and fat that were loosened during the bath. To prepare, squeeze the juice from half a lemon into warm bancha tea, or add one to two teaspoons of brown rice vinegar to bancha tea. Add a small, three-finger pinch of sea salt, stir, and use as a douche.

The hip bath and douche can be repeated twice a week for up to a month. During this time it is important to eat well and avoid the heavy fats, animal proteins, and simple sugars that have contributed to the condition.

Dried Daikon Tea

While daikon leaves can be used for a hip bath, daikon root can be used to make several teas that help melt fibroids. Fresh daikon has a strong yin or expansive effect and a person can become weak after taking it for several days. Dried daikon is stronger than fresh daikon and can be used for a longer period of time. Several years ago I introduced Dried Daikon Tea. It is good for dissolving all fatty substances, including those in fibroids and ovarian cysts. A small cup can be taken daily for two to three months.

Dried daikon can be made at home from the roots in your garden or purchased at natural food stores. Often it is sold shredded in packages imported from Japan. To prepare Dried Daikon Tea:

1. Combine 1 part dried, shredded daikon to 4 parts wa-

ter.

2. Bring to a boil, reduce flame, and simmer 15-30 minutes.

3. Toward the end of cooking, add a pinch of sea salt or several drops of shoyu, and let simmer until done.

This tea can also be prepared with lotus root, shiitake mushroom, and a small piece of kombu sea vegetable. The shiitake helps dissolve fat and protein deposits, while the kombu adds minerals and counters the strong expansive effects of the daikon and shiitake.

Chapter 4
PMS is Not PMS
By Helen Farrell, M.D.

Dr. Farrell is a physician practicing in Canada. This article is excerpted from the book, Doctors Look at Macrobiotics, *edited by Michio Kushi, Japan Publications, 1988.*

The premenstrual syndrome [PMS] is the cluster of symptoms that occurs from one to fourteen days before the onset of menses. The symptoms can be both physical and psychological. While the symptoms may vary from month to month as a woman reacts to the stresses of her personal life, family and work environments, they generally remain the same over a number of cycles. There is usually dramatic relief from the symptoms with the onset of the menstrual flow or at least within the first few days. In my practice I have found that women of all ages can have these problems from puberty until well after the menopause. It is more common, however, in the woman in her thirties.

When I lecture on PMS, I usually begin by describing what I consider to be a normal menstrual cycle, since many women are unaware of what is normal and what is not. And, historically speaking, women seem to have accepted the fact that they must grin and bear the monthly discomfort. The length of the cycle should be regular, plus or minus two to three days, and roughly 25 to 35 days in length. On day one, the onset of menstruation, there should be no discomfort or cramps. The flow should start immediately, a continuous red flow with no clots. The flow should subside completely within three to five days. At ovulation there may be a mucus discharge, and a few twinges in the right or left lower abdominal area. The moods should not be out of control. About five to seven days before the period, there may be slight water retention and a decrease in energy.

One of the most common complaints women have is premenstrual mood swings. Most women tell me that they can cope with the numerous physical discomforts, but it is the psychological symptoms that upset them and their families the most. At ovulation many women feel as though a switch has suddenly been turned on and they can no longer control their emotions. They become weepy, irritable, angry, irrational, uncoordinated, tired, short-fused, and possibly even suicidal.

It is obvious that the hormonal influence is a big factor in the severity of these symptoms. Estrogen and progesterone are known to alter the glucose-insulin metabolism thereby causing potential hypoglycemia. If the diet contains food or beverages that lower the blood sugar, this adds further to the problem. The extreme fluctuation in blood sugar prevents the brain from getting the constant supply of glucose it needs and consequently the "animal brain" takes over. This can account for many of the above symptoms.

If we are under stress (and women are under stress in the premenstrual phase) and consume sugar, then this causes changes in certain brain hormones which can produce nervous tension and fatigue. In addition, sugar and caffeine also trigger insulin release in excess of what the body needs, and the blood sugar subsequently drops. A lot of patients think that sugar gives them the energy they need to get through the day. It does, in fact, steal their energy away. Michelle Harrison, in her book, *Self-Help for Premenstrual Syndrome*, sums it up very well by saying that burning sugar for fuel is like using newspaper for heat—it burns easily with a bright flame then quickly dies out and you need more paper.

Therefore, by eliminating caffeine, sugar and other sweeteners, and eating small, frequent meals, the blood sugar can be stabilized. The mood swings are not as severe then. I have noted, however, that in some patients the mood swings do not disappear with dietary control. In these cases, I assume that external stresses, or perhaps underlying emotional problems are severe and consistent enough to trigger the premenstrual problems. It makes good sense, also, to schedule stressful events for other times in the cycle.

A woman may need about 500 calories a day more during the premenstrual phase. This means a general appetite increase. It does not mean specific food cravings. Because the North American diet is unbalanced and extreme, food cravings are common. Sugar cravings—and particularly chocolate cravings—are among the most common complaints in my practice. On a diet high in sugar, women will usually crave it more at a time when the blood glucose is low.

In macrobiotic theory, food cravings are explained by the overconsumption of extreme foods, that is, foods that are either too expansive or too contractive. If a contractive food is eaten, such as meat, cheese, or salt, the body will automatically crave expansive foods such as sugar to reestablish balance. This phenomenon is enhanced premenstrually when the glucose metabolism is altered.

Bloating is a problem most women experience. A typical North American diet can cause constant bloating. I consider a small amount of bloating as normal premenstrual physiology. However, if bloating is excessive, it can lead to headaches, irritability, dizziness, hypersensitivity to light, lethargy, swollen extremities, and a general feeling of discomfort. Water retention is frequently caused by the overconsumption of salt. In addition, a diet high in refined carbohydrates triggers insulin release which prevents the kidneys from excreting salt. This also contributes to water retention. Therefore, when patients cut down on their salt and sugar intake, the bloating is less.

Another bad habit patients have is consuming copious amounts of water. Of course, we constantly read about the health benefits of drinking a lot of water daily. But it stands to reason that if a person consumes six to eight glasses of water a day, plus tea, coffee, and juices, and bloating is a problem, then perhaps the kidneys cannot handle the load. The excess fluid is then deposited in the tissues. A lot of women urinate frequently and have to get up several times at night. This adds further stress at a time when it should be minimized.

Sore, swollen, lumpy breasts, beginning at ovulation and continuing until the menstrual flow, are a very common problem. In fact, in my practice, I estimate that 90 percent of my patients have tender breasts before their periods. For some patients this causes extreme discomfort. I used to use primrose oil and vitamin E for patients with the problem and noted a modest degree of success. However, it has become clear to me over the past few years that if women eliminate dairy products from their diet, breast problems disappear within two to three months.

Annemarie Colbin, in her book, *Food and Healing*, indicates that the consumption of dairy products appears to be strongly linked not only to breast discomfort, but also to other disorders of the female reproductive system such as ovarian tumors, cysts, vaginal discharge, infections, menstrual cramps, and heavy flow. She indicates that by eliminating foods that relate to the reproductive system of animals, such as milk and milk products, eggs, and the meat of animals raised on estrogens, the problems disappear.

Another frequent complaint is headaches. Premenstrual headaches are extremely common and seem to be associated with water retention, fatigue, and stress. I have found that the elimination of dairy foods from the diet has been one of the most important factors in alleviating migraine headaches. It is also essential to reduce water-retaining foods as well as those causing hypoglycemia. A lot of patients wake up with headaches. This group seems to experience unusual drops in blood sugar during the night. By reducing caffeine, sugar, and other sweeteners and by eating complex carbohydrates, this problem can be alleviated.

Most people I see tend to be constipated and have a history of hemorrhoids or other bowel dysfunction. "If the bowels don't work properly, then nothing else will" has been one of my favorite expressions for some time. I usually explain to my patients that the bowels are like a central processing unit. Everything that goes into the body is processed there. If they do not operate properly, then the body cannot assimilate the nutrients it needs on a regular basis. A lot of people use laxatives or add fiber to their diet. Bran is the "in thing" these days. Why not eat the whole grain instead of just parts of it?

The other common cause of constipation is the overconsumption of dairy products. Once patients eliminate these from their diet, they have regular and more frequent bowel movements. It is the mucus from dairy products that interferes with bowel function, causing constipation, diarrhea, gas, bloating, and hemorrhoids. Poor bowel function is also related to poor skin.

Most people do not understand the connections among the various systems of the body. They treat themselves, as does the majority of the medical profession, as a disconnected assortment of symptoms and problems. I have always suspected that the skin directly reflects what goes on inside the body. I am amused at a dermatologist's approach to skin disorders. While they may notice a modest success in their treatments, they completely ignore the internal state of affairs. Macrobiotics has certainly helped me understand the physiology associated with poor skin and the distribution of markings, pimples, and blemishes. I generally tell my patients that poor skin is a reflection of what goes on in the gastrointestinal tract and is therefore directly related to what goes into the mouth. There is no doubt about the connection between sugar intake and pimples. But I have also recently discovered, through macrobiotic readings, that the elimination of animal protein, along with sugar, clears up the skin remarkably well. It is interesting to note that when patients start to alter their diets, their skin can become worse during the first few months. I presume this is the discharge phase or "healing crisis."

Most women note a few pimples around the mouth or chin area before a period. This is understandable, since, in Oriental diagnosis, this area represents the reproductive organs. Again, this illustrates how hormones can intensify biochemical imbalances.

It is worthwhile mentioning the menopause here because, as with PMS, the symptoms associated with this time of life are merely a reflection of the poor nutritional status of a woman's body. Menopause is a natural event. If this is so, why do so many women suffer for years with numerous complaints? With the change in the ovaries, the decrease in hormone production, and the associated physiological changes, it is a great internal stress. It stands to reason, then, if the body is already operating in a compromised condition, any added stress is going to cause symptoms to appear. Therefore, the symptoms of menopause are like those of PMS, and this means that we deal with them in exactly the same way—with diet modification.

I see teenagers with the same problems that women have in their thirties and forties. It is sad that a lot of young girls suffer with severe menstrual cramps, vomiting, dizziness, and headaches, and miss one to two days of school every month. In addition, they may have poor skin, fatigue, and mood swings. The effect of poor nutrition seems to manifest itself at puberty, a time when there is great internal change or stress.

It was a patient who first introduced me to macrobiotics. I had heard the term before but really did not know too much about it. She suggested some books, and since at this time I was personally interested in improving my eating habits, I was anxious to learn more. My first macrobiotic book was *Introducing Macrobiotic Cooking* by Wendy Esko. Reading the introductory chapters was very enlightening. It all made so much sense to me. Having had medical training and the opportunity to see and talk to hundreds of patients about their bodies, I knew that I had to read more on this subject. Then I read Michio Kushi's books, *Natural Healing through Macrobiotics* and *How to See Your Health*, and a whole new world of medicine opened up for me.

I not only began applying some of my new-found knowledge to my patients, but I also began to cook macrobiotic foods for myself. Although my diet had not been totally unhealthy up to this point, my eating habits were somewhat erratic and I did have sugar binges. After one month of eating macrobiotic food and stopping my vitamins, I felt worse than I had for a long time. I got a bad cold and was physically and mentally run down. Of course, this was all part of the discharge and healing phase, but I had a difficult time understanding this concept then and the fact that the food-preparation time did not fit into my schedule sent me slowly back to my old eating habits.

Over the past year and a half, along with my continued reading, and applying macrobiotics to patient care, I have become convinced that this type of approach to nutrition was the one that not only I, but everyone else, should be following. After taking cooking classes and attending a macrobiotic conference, I have become a lot more organized in my approach to this way of eating and lifestyle. I have been more effective also in helping my patients make dietary adjustments based on my own experiences.

I have come a long way professionally and personally in my approach to PMS and other related problems. I used to believe that the only real cure for PMS was pregnancy. Naturally, the cyclical occurrence of symptoms disappears during pregnancy. However, there about thirty to forty hormones secreted at that time that can often mask the fact that the body is biochemically out of balance to start with. The pregnancy will add greater stress to the body and most likely make symptoms worse later on when the periods return.

PMS is not PMS. It is not a disease or a syndrome. It is merely a collection or focus of symptoms that occur in the female body as a result of stress, especially nutritional stress. Although some women have found vitamin therapy to be temporarily helpful, it is not a fundamental solution. The elimination or at least the decrease in the consumption of caffeine, refined salt, sugar, alcohol, dairy products, and meat helps everyone increase their vitality and decrease their symptoms regardless of what they may be, and can serve as a preliminary step toward more complete dietary change.

In our society today, many women find it difficult to make dietary adjustments, particularly when their families resist the change. If they can at least become more aware of how the food they eat affects their mind and body, then they will have taken a big step forward in achieving an optimal menstrual cycle and good health.

Chapter 5
Healthy Pregnancy
by Wendy Esko

Wendy Esko, a macrobiotic cooking teacher and author, is the mother of eight. This article was published in Macrobiotics Today, *March/April, 1992.*

Before my first pregnancy, I had heard little about the natural process of having children, except from several friends who had delivered their babies by natural childbirth. I often wondered what it was actually like to have a baby. In modern society, few women speak to each other about the actual experience of having children.

When I became pregnant for the first time, I began to wonder about things such as what kind of changes I would go through, what labor was like, how having a baby would change my life, and other questions. I had the feeling that every woman probably asked herself the same questions when she first became pregnant. I began to look for books on pregnancy and natural childbirth. Of course I realized that no person or book could answer all of my questions or teach me how to be a mother or have a baby. Although others can offer guidance based on their experiences, every new mother has to learn these things for herself.

One book that I found especially fascinating was *Biography of the Unborn* by Margaret Shea Gilbert. I first saw the book mentioned in the writings of George Ohsawa. It is short and simple and presents a month by month description of what a baby looks like during the stages of pregnancy, what kind of motions the developing baby is making, how and when the organs develop, and what kind of changes the mother's body is going through. It also describes the stages of labor. I found the book informative and easy to understand. It is written in a very charming style that conveys the author's sense of wonder at the miracle of life.

In Japan, there is a practice known as *Tai-Kyo*, or "embryonic education." The teaching of Tai-Kyo deals with the environment that surrounds a woman during pregnancy. Women were advised to read religious or spiritual books during pregnancy, and to try to cultivate respect and appreciation for life, beauty, and nature. They were also advised to avoid upsetting or unpleasant influences or surroundings.

During my pregnancies, I was intuitively attracted to books such as the Bible, the Tao Teh Ching, and other philosophical and spiritual classics. I also enjoyed reading macrobiotic literature. One book that I found particularly enjoyable was *Monkey*, the classic folk novel of China. I also enjoyed reading books on art and nature, as well as fairy tales and children's stories. I was also attracted to drawing, and felt a strong desire to cook. I did not want to see movies that depicted violence or cruelty, and began to appreciate the beauty of nature. I enjoyed listening to classical music, and found it difficult to listen to rock 'n roll. I also found it difficult to ride on the trolley because of the crowds and noise. I became increasingly sensitive to all forms of vibration.

Pregnancy is a very beautiful experience. During my pregnancies, I was calm, happy, and kept busy. By busy I don't mean hard physical labor, but the normal activities of daily life. I believe a woman's strength and endurance increase dramatically during pregnancy. I found it very difficult not to be active or busy doing something. Everyday things like walking, cleaning house, cooking, and studying were a source of joy. I also found it satisfying to stay home and not travel during pregnancy. I enjoyed the security and tranquility of my home environment.

I discovered that it was important to eat well, but not rigidly, during pregnancy. I felt the need to create a strong center in my diet by preparing balanced macrobiotic meals every day. That made it much easier to manage the minor cravings I experienced. I also enjoyed eating brown rice on a regular basis, and found it helpful to prepare it in different ways, including in rice balls, sushi, fried rice, and soft cereal. Combining it with millet, barley, and other whole grains made it especially appealing.

I discovered how important it is not to be rigid or overly conceptual with your diet during pregnancy. If you have cravings, follow them as long as you chew well and are moderate in your intake. It is not wrong to desire foods that you don't normally eat. What is wrong is to make yourself unhappy by feeling guilty. If you have cravings for certain foods, try to find good quality substitutes. You may be surprised to discover that something else satisfies you just as much. I had no desire to eat strong animal food, dairy, or refined sugar during pregnancy. Occasional white meat fish, seasonal fruits, high quality sweeteners, and other whole natural foods satisfied whatever cravings I had.

One of the most important decisions we had to make was whether to give birth at home or in a hospital. I have given birth six times at home, once at a special birthing facility, and once in the hospital, in each case, without complications of any kind. If you have your baby in a hospital, make sure that your doctor and other members of the hospital staff are well informed about your wishes about medication. Now that natural childbirth is becoming more popular, most hospitals will comply with your wishes.

In some states, there are laws stating that a newborn must have silver nitrate put into its eyes to protect it from exposure to venereal disease. However, for healthy mothers who are eating well, this is unnecessary.

If you have your baby at home, make sure that your doctor or midwife is aware of your wishes about medication. Most doctors who deliver at home will not give you or your baby routine medication if you insist that you don't wish to have it. I recommend that a doctor or experienced midwife be present at home births. If your body is not totally flexible, you may tear during delivery. Tearing is due to rigidity in the muscles caused by consumption of animal food in the past. During delivery, if you wait to push until you absolutely feel you have to push, there is less danger of tearing. If tearing does occur, you normally don't feel it, so don't worry. If you do tear and need to be stitched, it is often not necessary to have an anesthetic, as long as you breathe as you did during contractions. It is better to have stitches because they allow healing to occur more quickly and make it less likely for scar tissue to develop. Of course, every woman is different and must make these decisions for herself. I can only offer suggestions based on my experience.

I am fortunate to have not had medication (including anesthetics) during any of my deliveries, nor have any of my children had silver nitrate. I wanted my children to have the best start in life with no drugs of any kind.

I didn't feel that it was necessary to attend classes to learn how to breathe, exercise, or have a baby. If your are healthy, your breathing will come very naturally without having to force it. In my case, I was unable to force myself to do anything that I felt uncomfortable with. Of course, every woman is different and is free to decide for herself whether or not to attend classes or workshops on natural birthing.

My husband and I both agreed that he would not be in the room during the birth of our children. We both felt that his presence in the delivery room would be distracting, and that his not being present during birth would help maintain attraction. We also decided against having our older children in the room. However, I did find it comforting to have other women in the delivery room. As with all matters pertaining to pregnancy and birth, this is something for couples to decide for themselves.

Before your first child is born, it is hard to imagine what a great responsibility it is to have a baby. Our children are the key to the future. It is essential that we give them the best start in life.

Chapter 6
Menopause and Diet
By Edward Esko

The essence of life is change. Like everything in nature, women and men pass through stages in their growth and development. Menopause is one of these natural transitions. As with puberty and childbirth, menopause is a normal stage in a woman's life. In the modern world, however, there is a tendency to turn the natural processes of life into medical events. Such is the case with menopause.

Aging is the opposite of growth. Growth is yin or expansive, while aging is the process in which things become yang or contracted. During menopause, a woman becomes physically more yang. At the same time, her yin, invisible nature—in other words, her wisdom and spirituality—become deeper and richer.

During menopause, a woman produces less estrogen and progesterone, the primary female hormones. With that, menstruation gradually becomes less regular and eventually stops. If a woman is naturally healthy, these changes occur smoothly, and the transition through menopause is not accompanied by uncomfortable symptoms. However in today's world, dietary and lifestyle habits are causing many women to experience a variety of unnecessary symptoms during menopause.

The menstrual cycle is a beautiful example of harmony and balance. Menstruation is initiated by hormones produced by the pituitary gland located at the base of the brain. These hormones, known as follicle-stimulating hormone (FSH) and luteinizing hormone (LH) are strongly charged by yang energy spiraling down from the cosmos. This contracting force, known as heaven's force, enters the body at the top of the head. Heaven's energy charges the spiral center at the crown of the head as well as the region around the mid-brain, including the pituitary. As a result, pituitary hormones are strongly charged with heaven's contracting energy.

The lower body is complementary and opposite to the head. It is strongly charged by energy coming up from the earth. The ovaries and uterus are located in the lower body and receive a strong charge of earth's yin expanding force. When the pituitary produces FSH and LH, the ovaries respond by producing eggs. When an egg is produced, it sends out hormonal messages that tell the pituitary to reduce the production of FSH and LH. Yin counteracts and neutralizes yang. At menopause, the ovaries no longer produce eggs, and the pituitary keeps producing these hormones without the usual counteracting effect. This causes the level of these hormones in the blood to increase. At menopause, therefore, a woman's condition naturally becomes more yang or contracted.

Symptoms During Menopause

Studies of women in Japan, China, and other parts of the world where grains and other plant foods comprise the mainstay of the diet, show that they experience far fewer menopausal symptoms than women in the West. The Japanese, in fact, have no word in their language for "hot flashes." These studies, in addition to the many cases of symptom-free menopause experienced by macrobiotic and vegetarian women, suggest that a plant-based diet reduces, if not eliminates, many of the symptoms of menopause.

The principle of yin and yang can help us understand why some women experience no symptoms at menopause, while others experience many. As we saw above, menopause is a time when a woman naturally becomes more yang. If her diet is based on vegetable quality foods which counteract the effects of strong yang, then she can more easily pass through menopause without symptoms. If, however, her diet includes plenty of meat, eggs, chicken, cheese, and other strongly yang animal foods, her condition becomes unbalanced and she will be more likely to develop symptoms.

A review of the common symptoms of menopause suggests they are part of an overall syndrome resulting primarily from an overly yang or contracted condition.

Hot Flashes At least three-quarters of American women experience hot flashes during menopause. During a hot flash, heat and energy are discharged. A woman experiences a feeling of heat (her skin temperature increases), followed by a period of sweating. In some cases, hot flashes interrupt sleep, producing symptoms of sleep deprivation such as mood swings, fatigue, and chronic irritation. Hot flashes occur when excess energy builds up inside the body. This excess gathers toward the center of the body and is suddenly discharged outward toward the periphery. The most common dietary sources of this excess are foods such as chicken, cheese, eggs, meat, and high-fat fish such as tuna and salmon.

Up until menopause, the female hormones (estrogen and progesterone) help counteract excess yang in the body. However, at menopause, the decline in these hormones makes it easier for excess to accumulate, leading to hot flashes and other symptoms.

Vaginal Dryness and Thinning The lining of the vagina consists of many layers of cells. Those at the surface are the most yin and most dependent upon estrogen and other female hormones. When hormone levels fall, the outermost layer of cells—about six cells thick—often becomes depleted. Thinning of the vaginal lining produces symptoms such as dryness, itching, and pain during intercourse. In some cases the yin, outermost cells of the urethra also become thinner, leading to frequent urination.

The dietary cause of this condition is the repeated consumption of eggs, chicken, meat, cheese, and other animal products, together with too much salt and foods high in sodium. The repeated intake of foods high in saturated fat and cholesterol causes a layer of hard fat to build up just below the surface of the vagina. These deposits interfere with the flow of moisture and oils to the surface, resulting in dryness and constriction. Too many baked flour products, such as cookies, bread, crackers, and chips, also contribute to an overly dry condition.

Vaginal dryness is not unlike the drying and hardening of the skin that occurs following years of eating plenty of animal food. When the skin becomes dry and tight, excess energy no longer discharges through the normal channels. Hot flashes are one way in which this accumulated energy is discharged from the body. A macrobiotic diet, which is low in fat and cholesterol, can prevent excessive dryness from occurring, both at the surface of the body and in the vagina.

Mood Swings and Depression These symptoms are primarily the result of low blood sugar, or hypoglycemia. The hormonal changes that occur at menopause exacerbate blood sugar imbalances. Hypoglycemia is related to the condition of the pancreas, the organ that regulates blood sugar. Normally, blood sugar is maintained in balance by the pancreatic hormones insulin and glucagon. Insulin cause the blood sugar to drop, while glucagon causes it to rise. Insulin is strongly charged with yang, contracting energy, while glucagon is charged with yin, expansive force. If the pancreas is healthy, these hormones function appropriately and the person's blood sugar stays within the normal range.

However, in many cases, repeated consumption of strong contractive foods such as chicken, cheese, and eggs causes the pancreas to become hard and tight. The cells that secrete glucagon become tight and constricted and their output is reduced. When this happens, the blood sugar tends to stay below normal, causing the person to crave sugar, fruit, alcohol, coffee or other stimulants in an attempt to raise it. The brain is especially sensitive to fluctuations in blood sugar and when there is a deficit, a person's moods tend to be depressed or down. Simple sugars or stimulants have only a temporary effect. A person must continually take them in order to lift his or her mood, and they cause a steady depletion in the person's energy as a whole.

Some women experience a lack of clear thinking during menopause. This condition is known as "fuzzy thinking" and is primarily due to hypoglycemia. Low blood sugar deprives the brain of the glucose it needs for optimal functioning, resulting in a loss of clarity. Sugar or alcohol, which are often used to relieve hypoglycemia, further interfere with mental clarity. They also produce extreme emotional fluctuations. As with the symptoms described above, hypoglycemia and mood disorders are primarily the result of the repeated intake of animal food.

Long-Term Symptoms

The long-term symptoms associated with menopause are consistent with the repeated consumption of meat, dairy, and other animal foods, or in other words, a diet based on too many yang extremes. These symptoms include the following.

Osteoporosis It is well known that countries with the highest intakes of meat and dairy have the highest rates of osteoporosis. (The highest rates of osteoporosis are found among the Eskimo, who eat a diet comprised almost entirely of animal food.) Countries with a low intake of meat and dairy, and a high intake of grains, vegetables, and other plant fibers, have low rates of this disease. Women who consume a modern meat- and dairy-centered diet are therefore at high risk for osteoporosis. Because of their diet, many American women experience up to a two to five percent loss of bone during menopause, with some degree of bone loss continuing after menopause.

Although female hormones play a role in the health of the bones, the loss of bone often begins prior to menopause, an indication that long-term dietary and lifestyle factors are just as important as the decline in estrogen at menopause. Estrogen, which is yin, prevents bone loss, while progesterone, which is slightly more yang, stimulates the formation of bone. In the macrobiotic view, bone loss results from extremes of either yin or yang. The high consumption of meat, dairy, and other animal foods (yang) causes an over-acid condition in the blood. In order to neutralize this acid, the body mobilizes calcium and other minerals from the bones. The saturated fat found in these foods reduces the absorption of calcium from the diet, thus compounding the problem.

Sugar, soft drinks, and other yin extremes also produce an acid reaction in the blood that leads to a similar mobilization of calcium and bone loss. Phosphorous also produces an acid reaction and foods high in this element, such as soda and red meat, promote osteoporosis. Alcohol and caffeine (extreme yin) also promote loss of calcium, as does cigarette smoking and consumption of too much salt (extreme yang).

As we saw above, desire for alcohol and caffeine arises as a result of hypoglycemia. Low blood sugar triggers the desire for sugar or stimulants that cause a temporary rise in blood sugar. Cigarettes or salty snacks are often taken to balance the intake of coffee, sweets, and alcohol, thus setting in motion a pattern that leads to a progressive loss of calcium. Along with diet, lack of exercise contributes to bone loss.

Avoidance of meat, dairy, chicken, and other animal foods makes it easier to stay away from sugar, soft drinks, and caffeine. A balanced macrobiotic diet based on whole grains, beans, fresh vegetables, sea vegetables, and other whole natural foods, many of which are high in calcium, in combination with a normally active lifestyle, can help prevent osteoporosis while safeguarding the health of the bones.

Heart Disease It is well established that the modern epidemic of heart disease is primarily a function of the modern high-fat diet and sedentary lifestyle rather than a function of diminished hormone levels at menopause. Epidemiological and other studies support the role of a diet high in meat, eggs, chicken, cheese, and other animal products in causing high cholesterol levels and an elevated risk of heart attack and related cardiovascular problems. Conversely, numerous studies support the role of a balanced grain- and vegetable-based diet in preventing and reversing heart disease.

Because it is yin, estrogen counteracts the yang factors (arising primarily from repeated consumption of animal food) that lead to heart disease. One National Institute of

Health study showed that women taking estrogen or an estrogen-progesterone combination had lower cholesterol levels and clotting factors than women not taking hormone replacement. Strong yin (synthetic estrogen) counteracts the buildup of hard fatty deposits in the blood vessels. Aspirin and other cholesterol-lowering drugs, also strongly yin, have a similar effect. However, both hormone replacement therapy and cholesterol drugs have potential side effects. Changing to a grain- and vegetable-based diet can help women reduce their risk of heart disease without side effects.

Natural Hormone Replacement

Hormone replacement therapy (HRT), in which synthetic or naturally-derived hormones are given to women during and after menopause, has now become a routine part of medical practice. An estimated 40 percent of menopausal women in the United States are using HRT. Premarin, an estrogen replacement made from the urine of pregnant mares, is used by more than 8 million American women, making it the most popular drug in the U.S. Hormone creams and patches are being used by millions of more women.

Even though it is used by millions of women, synthetic HRT has its drawbacks. Several studies have linked synthetic HRT with an increased risk of breast and endometrial cancer. Synthetic HRT can produce a variety of other side effects. As we saw above, estrogen is strongly yin or expansive. Synthetic HRT is an extreme answer to symptoms caused by an extreme diet, especially too many animal foods. HRT does not change the cause of these symptoms; it merely counteracts them while producing side effects of its own.

Natural hormone replacement, such as that utilizing the naturally-occurring progesterone in Mexican yams, soybeans, and other botanicals is certainly less extreme than synthetic hormone replacement. However, natural hormone replacement without dietary change does not address the root cause of the problem. Even though it may help relieve symptoms, it is not a fundamental solution. It is probably for that reason that advocates of natural progesterone therapy, such as John Lee, M.D., also recommend a grain- and vegetable-based diet.

Phytoestrogens

The most ideal situation occurs when a woman manages her hormone balance through her daily diet. Recent studies have shown that grains, beans, and traditional soyfoods such as tofu and miso contain phytoestrogens (phtyo = plant); mild estrogen-like compounds. Phytoestrogens help relieve symptoms caused by hormone deficiency. Soybeans are also a source of natural progesterone.

Phytoestrogens can lower the risk of breast and endometrial cancer, both of which are linked to high estrogen levels in the body. Mild phytoestrogens and the pathological estrogens that accelerate female cancers are both yin. Phytoestrogens are mildly yin, while pathological estrogens are extremely yin. (Pathological estrogens are accelerated by the intake of milk, ice cream, sugar, and chocolate, as well as by foods such as chicken, turkey, beef, and others treated with synthetic growth hormones.) Since likes repel, phytoestrogens cause pathological estrogens to be excreted from the body. The higher the intake of foods rich in phytoestrogens, the greater the excretion of pathological estrogens. This may help explain the relatively low rates of breast cancer among Chinese and Japanese women. Asian women regularly consume miso, tofu, and other foods containing phytoestrogens.

Nabé and Other Tofu Dishes

Tofu has cooling and relaxing effects and can be helpful in relieving hot flashes. It can be lightly cooked with vegetables, or in severe cases, occasionally eaten raw with a pinch of grated ginger, chopped fresh scallion, and several drops of shoyu. Tofu also contains calcium, and when eaten with other calcium-rich foods, such as green leafy vegetables, sea vegetables (especially hiziki and arame), beans, and seeds, as a part of a balanced macrobiotic diet, can help prevent osteoporosis. The following dish, known as Yuki Nabé, is made with grated daikon and fresh tofu, and can be used to ease hot flashes and other menopausal symptoms.

Clay Nabé pots are available at natural and Oriental food stores and through mail order. They can be used to prepare a variety of vegetable dishes. Yuki Nabé is made from grated daikon and tofu, and has a pure white color. Hence the the name Yuki Nabé , which means "pot of snow." If you cannot find a Nabé pot, prepare the dish in a stainless steel or enamel pot with a lid.

Ingredients and Utensils:

1 1/2 cup fresh daikon radish
1/3 cup tofu
pinch of sea salt
small or medium Nabé pot (a small stainless or enamel
   pot can be used instead)
vegetable grater (for fine grating)
Japanese-style vegetable knife

Preparation:

1. Peel and grate daikon.
2. Place grated daikon in Nabé pot.
3. Add a small pinch of sea salt.
4. Cover and place on a medium flame.
5. Cook for 3 to 5 minutes.
6. Slice tofu into cubes.
7. Place in Nabé pot with grated daikon.
8. Cover and cook for 3 to 5 minutes (until tofu is done.)
9. Remove cover and serve.

Yuki Nabé can be eaten by itself, with brown rice, or as part of a meal. Yuki Nabé has a delicious sweet flavor and doesn't require additional seasoning. The Nabé pot serves a dual function. It is used to cook the dish and also to serve it. Simply remove the Nabé from the burner and place it on your table with a pot-holder under it.

When cooked in this way, daikon and tofu become sweet. Yuki Nabé helps melt stagnation (just like melting snow), relax inner tension, and establish active energy flow. It can be included several times per week.

Sweet Vegetable Drink

The mood swings that accompany menopause can be remedied by basing the diet on complex carbohydrates, especially naturally sweet foods such as whole grains (including sweet brown rice and mochi), and sweet vegetables (such as squash, pumpkin, cabbage, carrots, and onions). Naturally sweet desserts, such as chestnut purees, rice, sweet rice, squash, and amasake puddings, and cooked fruit desserts, occasionally sweetened with rice syrup or barley malt, help ease hypoglycemia and mood swings.

Sweet vegetables provide a readily available source of complex carbohydrates that can help relieve mood swings and other symptoms of hypoglycemia. They may be eaten regularly, or taken in the more concentrated form of sweet vegetable drink. To prepare this special drink, cut equal amounts of carrots, squash (select those with an orange color on the inside), onions, and green cabbage into very fine pieces. Place the cut vegetables in a pot with four times as much water, cover, and bring to a boil. Reduce the flame to low and simmer for 15 to 20 minutes. Remove from the stove and strain the liquid through a fine mesh strainer into a large glass jar.

The strained liquid—or "sweet vegetable drink"—can be stored in the refrigerator for several days. One or two cups can be taken daily or several times per week depending on the severity of the condition. Sweet vegetable drink may be continued for a month or so or until the symptoms of hypoglycemia improve. To serve, heat in a saucepan until warm, or let it sit for several minutes until it becomes room temperature.

Body Scrubbing

A plant-based macrobiotic diet is low in saturated fat and cholesterol, and helps restore normal moisture and flexibility to the skin, including the lining of the vagina. The regular use of high-quality sesame oil in sauteing can help naturally moisturize the skin. The daikon hip bath described in Michio Kushi's chapter on "Fibroids and Reproductive Health" can also be used to restore a moisture and flexibility to the vaginal lining.

Daily body scrubbing with a hot wet towel also helps open the pores while melting away hard fat deposits that interfere with the flow of moisture to the surface. It helps prevent drying of the skin and the buildup of energy that can produce hot flashes. Body scrubbing can be done before or after a bath or shower, or anytime. It takes only about ten minutes to do. All you need is a sink with hot water and a medium-sized cotton bath towel. Hold the towel at either end and place the center of the towel under the stream of hot water. Wring out the towel, and while it is still hot and steamy begin to scrub with it. Do a section of the body at a time. For example, begin with the hands and fingers and work your way up the arms to the shoulders, neck, and face, then down to the chest, upper back, abdomen, lower back, buttocks, legs, feet, and toes. Scrub until the skin becomes slightly red or until each part becomes warm. Reheat the towel by running it under hot water after doing each section or as soon as it starts to cool. A body scrub can be done first thing in the morning, before going to bed, or at both times of the day. Aside from softening and energizing the skin, the body scrub helps dissolve tension and stress and brighten your mood.

Women who eat macrobiotically have cholesterol levels that are below the normally high averages in the United States and other Western nations. (In studies of macrobiotic people conducted by researchers at Harvard University and elsewhere, the average cholesterol level was found to be 125 mg/dl.) Women with high cholesterol who change to a macrobiotic diet often experience a rapid drop in their cholesterols within several weeks. Clearly, macrobiotic eating can prevent and even reverse heart disease.

A diet based on whole natural foods is the cornerstone of a healthy, symptom-free menopause. When she is free of unnecessary symptoms, menopause can be a happy time in which a woman's spirituality and consciousness develop toward deeper and richer levels.

Chapter 7
Healthy Bones and Teeth
by Gale Jack

When I was younger, I occasionally came across the word "osteoporosis" in my reading but never paid much attention to it. I always associated it with older people. So I was totally unprepared when a dentist turned away from my X-rays and said, "You have the most advanced case of osteoporosis I've ever seen in a woman your age!"

Unfortunately, my experience may not be that uncommon. Many women may have osteoporosis and not know it until they've fractured a hip or wrist or have been told that they have to have dentures because of extensive bone loss. X-rays do not appear to be sensitive enough to detect bone deterioration until 30 percent of the bone mass is lost.

Osteoporosis is the thinning and loss of bone tissue which leaves the body subject to fracture and falls and loss of supporting structures of the teeth. In extreme cases, it can cause spinal collapse, recurrent back pain, and "dowager's hump," a hump on the upper back most frequently seen in older women where the upper spine curves outward, the lower spine curves inward, and the stomach protrudes. And osteoporosis can precipitate hip fractures in elderly women which leads to death in 30 percent of those injured.

An estimated 200,000 osteoporotic American women over the age of forty-five fracture one or more of their bones annually. Of these, 40,000 die of complications following their injuries.

Loss of bone begins sooner and proceeds more rapidly in women than in men. It affects 25 percent of women after a natural meopause (with the most rapid bone loss occurring the five to six years following menopause) and up to 50 percent of those who have had a surgical menopause (brought about by the removal of ovaries or the uterus or both). Small body size, independent of body weight, is a critical risk factor.

Women of all sizes seem to have more bone loss than men and have it an an earlier age, but they are not the only ones affected. Michio Kushi estimates that between 60 and 70 percent of all people in modern society suffer from osteoporosis.

It's certainly much more widespread than is revealed by medical statistics because there are few outward signs of the disease in the early stages.

One sign is what's called transparent skin. If you can see the edges of both the large and small veins on the back of the hand then you may have osteoporosis as this reflects a lack of collagen in the skin's outer layers. One study of older women with osteoporosis showed that 83 percent had transparent skin while 13 percent did not.

Changes also are show up in the mouth, in the deterioration of tissues and bone surrounding and supporting the teeth. The earliest type of gum infection is known as gingivitis and is characterized by tenderness, swelling and bleeding of gum tissue. In more advanced cases, the gums may appear reddish blue or even deep blue showing that the blood has condensed and stagnated in those areas. Once pockets of infection occur between the teeth and gums where the gums have pulled away from the teeth, it's referred to as periodontal disease. At this stage, plaque accumulates on the teeth and keeps the gums from reattaching. The general view of dentists is that the infection leads to receding gums and the loss of bone that supports the teeth, causing the teeth to become loose. But I suspect the bone deterioration comes first, causing the receding gums and predisposing formation of the pockets as receding gum tissue parallels the loss of bone. After age thirty-five, the most common cause of tooth loss is periodontal disease.

The symptomatic treatment of advanced periodontitis

(where the gum tissues have receded beyond a certain level, plaque advances down the tooth roots and in some cases, a lack of bone density is present on X-rays of the mouth and some teeth may be loose) is extraction of the tooth or a mouthful of teeth, depending on the dentist and how many teeth he or she perceives as hopeless. The teeth may be perfectly sound, but in the medical view, the supporting tissues cannot sustain them so they simply extract them.

Periodontists (dentists who specialize in periodontal disease) may recommend scaling (removal of tartar from below the gum line), curettage (removing the degenerated, diseased soft tissue lining of the periodontal pocket using a local anesthesia), root planing (removing irregular surfaces along the root of the tooth), and polishing the teeth as corrective measures in less advanced cases of gum disease. In more chronic or advanced cases, the diseased gum tissue may be surgically removed and the exposed root surfaces scaled, the bones re-shaved, and gum tissues transplanted. None of these procedures address the cause and they can cause endless additional problems such as increased looseness and sensitivity in the teeth, further exposure of the tooth root, disturbance of the energy pathways in the meridians, and adverse reactions to anesthesia.

Physicians and macrobiotic teachers both understand that calcium and phosphorous are the major components of bone and when the amount of phosphorous is greater than the amount of calcium, bone loss occurs. But the medical profession would have us increase the intake of dairy products such as milk, cheese, and ice cream, along with canned seafoods (especially tuna, salmon, shrimp, and sardines), meat and poultry. In addition, calcium supplements are often recommended.

However, if that were effective in protecting the bones then I could never have developed osteoporosis because I ate plenty of all those foods for over thirty years. I had cheese, eggs, milk, meat, chicken, or tuna on a daily basis and later on added calcium supplements. And most people today eat plenty of meat and dairy foods. More recent studies show that excess protein actually increases calcium excretion and leads to overall loss of calcium from the body. (See the studies on diet and osteoporosis inthe Appendix.)

A diet of meat, poultry, eggs, milk, dairy, fish, simple sugar, chocolate, fruit, juice, and oily, greasy foods, along with few good quality whole grains and vegetables, creates an acidic condition in the blood so the body has to use the minerals stored in the bones to maintain an alkaline blood condition causing the bones to become weak. And if this diet is eaten for a prolonged period, then osteoporosis develops. On the other hand, whole grains, vegetables, sea salt, miso, soy sauce; beans cooked with sea salt, kombu, and root vegetables; bean products and sea vegetables, along with fresh organically grown vegetables, will create an alkaline blood condition. (Whole grains, if analyzed, become acid, but when we eat them, the phosphoric acids eliminate very yin factors in our body such as radiation so they, too, contribute to an alkaline blood condition.)

The macrobiotic way of eating not only prevents osteoporosis but it can remineralize bones that have been thinned. I saw one medically documented case in which this occurred. A woman from Atlanta followed the standard macrobiotic diet set forth by Michio Kushi, along with a few adjustments and way of life suggestiions. She had medical tests before seeing him and after about two years of macrobiotic practice. The latter tests showed that her bones had remineralized. They were at about 90 percent of maximum density.

There is no need for the macrobiotic woman (or man) to suffer fractures or have her teeth removed, even if she is told they are hopeless. But it is important to take cooking classes and practice well. If you are eating grains and vegetables, but take in too many baked flour products such as cookies, cakes, crackers, and hard bread or too much fruit, fruit juices, tofu cream pies, and amasake, you may not be successful. And even one doughnut or sugar-sweetened dessert per week can have a harmful effect on the teeth and bones. If you misuse salt by not cooking it into the foods of if you overuse salt, pickles, and condiments, you won't be able to stay away from sweets. But if you take care day by day, then you can have a long, happy life—free from osteoporosis.

Six years ago, a dentist looked at my X-rays and shook his head. He said I had to have full upper and lower dentures. None of my teeth could be saved. Fortunately, I didn't have the $3,000 he wanted for dentures, and I wasn't attracted by such extreme measures; by the time I could afford them, my understanding had improved somewhat.

Then during a recent busy period of my life during a cold Becket winter, I became too yang and corrected that condition with lots of barley malt-kuzu drinks (heavy on the barley malt!) and amasake which loosened one of my front teeth. I panicked and sought the opinion of several dentists. The third time I heard the same story—that my teeth couldn't be saved, I had no supporting bone—I gave in and had a number of upper teeth pulled.

It was a traumatic experience which proved to me how very precious our natural teeth are. After deep self-reflection and a return to a more balanced eating, I realized it was totally unnecessary to have had them pulled. Time, patience, and a few adjustments in my way of eating would have won out.

Osteoporosis is a silent threat only for those who don't understand the order of the universe or who refuse to live in harmony with it. For those who understand yin and yang, maintaining healthy bones and teeth may not be "a piece of cake," but it may begin with avoiding one.

Appendix
Scientific and Medical Research
on Women's Health
By Alex Jack

The following studies are summarized from Let Food Be Thy Medicine *by Alex Jack, One Peaceful World Press, a summary of 265 scientific and medical studies related to macrobiotics and holistic health.*

Soybeans and Breast Cancer
Scientists reported that a diet high in soybeans reduced the incidence of breast cancer in laboratory experiments. The active ingredient in the soybeans was identified as protease inhibitors, also found in certain other beans and seeds.

Source: W. Troll, "Blocking of Tumor Promotion by Protease Inhibitors," in J. H. Burchenal and H. F. Oettgen (eds.), *Cancer: Achievements, Challenges, and Prospects for the 1980s, Vol. 1,* New York: Grune and Stratton, pp. 549-55, 1980.

Estrogen and Breast Cancer
Macrobiotic and vegetarian women are less likely to develop breast cancer, researchers at New England Medical Center in Boston reported. The scientists found that macrobiotic and vegetarian women process estrogen differently from other women and eliminate it more quickly from their body. The study involved forty-five pre- and postmenopausal women, about half of whom were macrobiotic and vegetarian and half nonvegetarian. The women consumed about the same number of total calories. Although the vegetarian women took in only one third as much animal protein and animal fat, they excreted two to three times as much estrogen. High levels of estrogen have been associated with the development of breast cancer. "The difference in estrogen metabolism may explain the lower incidence of breast cancer in vegetarian women," the study concluded.

Source: B. R. Goldin et al., "Effect of Diet on Excretion of Estrogens in Pre- and Postmenopausal Incidence of Breast Cancer in Vegetarian Women," *Cancer Research* 41:3771-73, 1981.

Sea Vegetables and Breast Cancer

In an experiment at the Harvard School of Public Health, laboratory animals fed a control diet with 5 percent Laminaria (kombu), a brown sea vegetable, developed induced mammary cancer later than animals not fed seaweed. "Seaweed has shown consistent anti-tumor activity in several in vivo animal tests," the researcher concluded. "In extrapolating these results to the Japanese population, seaweed may be an important factor in explaining the low rates of certain cancers in Japan. Breast cancer shows a three-fold-lower rate among premenopausal Japanese women and a nine-fold-lower rate among postmenopausal women in Japan than reported for women in the United States. Since low levels of exposure to some toxic substances have been shown to be carcinogenic, then it may be that low levels of daily intake of food with antitumor properties may reduce cancer incidence."

Source: J. Teas, M. L. Harbison, and R. S. Gelman, "Dietary Seaweed [Laminaria] and Mammary Carcinogenesis in Rats," *Cancer Research* 44:2758-61, 1984.

Sea Vegetables and Breast Cancer

In Japan, tests on six groups of female rats showed that adding sea vegetables to the diet significantly inhibited induced mammary tumorigenesis. "Tumor incidences were 35 percent (7/20), 35 percent (7/20) and 50 percent (9/18), respectively [for groups fed nori, kombu, and another type of kombu], whereas that in the control group was 69 percent (920/29)," investigators reported. The onset of tumors was also delayed in the seaweed groups, and the weight of tumors was lower.

Source: Ichiro Yamamoto et al., "The Effect of Dietary Seaweeds on 7,12-Dimethyl-Benz[a]Anthracene-Induced Mammary Tumorigenesis in Rats," *Cancer Letters* 35:109-18, 1987.

Dairy and Breast Cancer

• Dairy food may be the most potent factor in the development of breast cancer. A study of 250 women with breast cancer in the northwestern province of Vercelli, Italy, found that they tended to consume considerably more milk, high-fat cheese, and butter than 499 healthy women of the same age in Italy and France.

Breast cancer risk tripled among women who consumed about half their calories as fat, 13 to 23 percent of their calories as saturated fat, and 8 to 20 percent of their calories as animal protein.

"These data suggest that during adult life, a reduction in dietary intake of fat and proteins of animal origin may contribute to a substantial reduction in the incidence of breast cancer in population subgroups with high intake of animal products," researchers concluded. "[A] diet rich in fat, saturated fat, or animal proteins may be associated with a twofold to threefold increase in a woman's risk of breast cancer."

Source: Paolo Toniolo et al., "Calorie-Providing Nutrients and Risk of Breast Cancer," *Journal of the National Cancer Institute* 81:278-86, 1989.

• In a Swiss case-control study, researchers found that breast cancer incidence was associated with higher consumption of meat, cheese, and alcohol, with cheese elevating risk the highest (2.7 times normal). Conversely, vegetable consumption offered significant protection (40 to 60 percent on average), especially green leafy vegetables.

Source: F. Levi et al., "Dietary Factors and Breast Cancer Risk in Vaud, Switzerland," *Nutrition and Cancer* 19:327-335, 1993.

Miso and Breast Cancer

The incidence of breast cancer in first-generation Japanese migrants to Hawaii is about 60 percent of the rate in subsequent generations of Japanese born in Hawaii. Researchers at the Departments of Nutrition Sciences and Biostatistics/Biomathematics, University of Alabama at Birmingham, theorized that miso, natto, soy sauce, and other traditionally fermented soybean foods may contribute to lowered disease. The consumption of these foods in Japan is about five times or more what it is among Japanese migrants to Hawaii.

To test their hypothesis, the scientists initiated feeding trials with rats and found that feeding miso to the rats delayed the appearance of induced breast cancer compared with animals on the control diet. The miso- and salt-supplemented diet treatment group showed a trend toward a lower number of cancers per animal, a trend toward a higher number of benign tumors per animal, and a trend toward a lower growth rate of cancers compared with controls.

"This data suggest that miso consumption may be a factor producing a lower breast cancer incidence in Japanese women," the researchers concluded. "Organic compounds found in fermented soybean-based foods may exert a chemoprotective effect."

Source: J. E. Baggott et al., "Effect of Miso (Japanese Soybean Paste) and NaCl on DMBA-Induced Rat Mammary Tumors," *Nutrition and Cancer* 14:103-09, 1990.

Tofu and Breast Cancer

British researchers reported in 1993 that natural phytoestrogens found in whole grains and soybean products, such as tofu, may protect against breast cancer. Professor Nick Day, director of the Institute for Public Health at Cambridge, explained that components found in these foods appeared to work in the same way as tamoxifen, a drug that has been used in conventional therapy.

"Certainly 50 grams of soya protein daily has a major effect on hormonal activity in premenopausal women," says Dr. Day. Tamoxifen has been associated with harmful side effects, while a diet high in tofu and whole grain products may prove as effective, he concluded. More research is planned as part of a European study.

Source: "Tofu May Be a Weapon Against Cancer," *London Times*, October 24, 1993.

Dairy and Ovarian Cancer

Dairy food consumption has been linked with ovarian cancer by researchers at Harvard. The scientists noted that women with ovarian cancer had low blood levels of transferase, an enzyme involved in the metabolism of dairy foods. The researchers theorized that women with low levels of transferase who eat dairy foods, especially yogurt and cottage cheese, could increase their risk of ovarian cancer by as much as three times.

The researchers estimated that women who consume large amounts of yogurt and cottage cheese increased their risk of ovarian cancer up to three times.

"Yogurt was consumed at least monthly by 49 percent of cases and 36 percent of controls," researchers reported. "World wide, ovarian cancer risk is strongly correlated with lactase persistence and per capita milk consumption, further epidemiological evidence that lactose rather than fat is the key dietary variable for ovarian cancer . . . [A]voidance of lactose-rich food by adults may be a way of primary prevention of ovarian cancer . . . "

Source: Daniel W. Cramer et al., "Galactose Consumption and Metabolism in Relation to the Risk of Ovarian Cancer," *Lancet* 2:66-71, 1989.

Green Vegetables and Female Cancers

European scientists reported that green vegetables were highly protective against ovarian cancer and endometrial cancer.

Source: C. La Vecchia et al., "Nutrition and Diet in the Etiology of Endometrial Cancer," *Cancer* 57: 1248-53, 1986.

Diet and Cervical Cancer

An Italian case-control study found that 191 women with invasive cervical cancer consumed less carrots and green vegetables than healthy women. Both foods were highly protective, with almost a fivefold increased risk associated with eating carrots less often than once a week or green vegetables less often than once a day.

Source: C. La Vecchia et al., "Dietary Vitamin A and the Risk of Invasive Cervical Cancer," *International Journal of Cancer* 34:319-22, 1984.

Diet and Lung Cancer

In a dietary study of women who never smoked cigarettes, researchers found that that those who consumed high amounts of vegetables, especially green and yellow vegetables high in carotene, had significantly lower risk of developing lung cancer than women who consumed fewer amounts of these foods.

Source: E. C. Candelora, "Dietary Intake and Risk of Lung Cancer in Women Who Never Smoked," *Nutrition and Cancer* 17:263-70, 1992.

Meat and Colon Cancer

Women who eat beef, lamb, or pork as a daily main dish are at two and a half times the risk for developing colon cancer as women who eat meat less than once a month. The conclusion, drawn from a study of 88,751 nurses, over a ten-year period, found that the more fish and poultry in the diet the less chances of getting colon cancer. "The substitution of other protein sources, such as beans or lentils, for red meat might also be associated with a reduced risk of colon cancer in populations that consume more legumes," researchers concluded. Investigators also found that eating the fiber from fruit appeared to reduce the risk of colon cancer. The fruits mentioned as possibly protective included apples and pears.

"The less red meat the better," recommended Dr. Walter Willett, professor of epidemiology and nutrition at the Harvard School of Public Health, who directed the study. "At most, it should be eaten only occasionally. And it may be maximally effective not to eat red meat at all."

Sources: Walter C. Willett et al., "Relation of Meat, Fat, and Fiber Intake to the Risk of Colon Cancer in a Prospective Study among Women," New England Journal of Medicine 323:1664-72, 1990 and Anastasia Toufexis, "Red Alert on Red Meat," *Time*, December 24, 1990.

Vitamin E and Colon Cancer

In a large prospective cohort study of 35,215 Iowa nurses, researchers found that women who consumed foods high in Vitamin E or took supplements high in this nutrient developed significantly less colon cancer. Vitamin E is high in whole grains, seeds and nuts, and other vegetable-quality foods.

Source: R. M. Bostick, "Reduced Risk of Colon Cancer with High Vitamin E: The Iowa Women's Health Study," *Cancer Research* September 13, 1993.

Premenstrual Syndrome (PMS)

• A survey found that women with anxiety symptoms associated with PMS, including nervous tension, mood swings, irritability, anxiety, and insomnia, ate two and a half times as much sugar as women without PMS or with mild cases. Dairy and caffeine intake have also been associated with PMS in other studies.

Source: G. E. Abraham, "Magnesium Deficiency in Premenstrual Tension," *Magnesium Bulletin* 1:68-73, 1982.

• MIT researchers reported that women consuming a diet high in complex carbohydrates and low in protein showed "improved depression, tension, anger, confusion, sadness, fatigue, alertness, and calmness" before the onset of menstruation in comparison to women with severe PMS eating the usual diet high in refined carbohydrates and fat. Besides sweets, the women suffering from PMS consumed more calories and more snack foods. Evidence was found that they intuitively tried to generate positive moods by ingesting more carbohydrates such as bread, rolls, and pasta and avoiding foods rich in protein.

Source: Judith J. Wurtman et al., "Effect of Nutrient Intake on Premenstrual Depression," *American Journal of Obstetrics and Gynecology* 161:1228-34, 1989.

• A new medical textbook on reproductive health and disorders recommends a high-fiber, low-fat diet to help prevent or reduce PMS. "Diet throughout the month, and especially during the premenstrual interval, should be high in complex carbohydrates and moderate in protein (emphasizing alternatives to red meat), but low in refined sugar and salt (sodium), with regular, small meals throughout the day." The authors further recommended that "women should reduce or eliminate their consumption of tea, coffee, caffeine-containing beverages, chocolate, and alcohol, and stop smoking."

Source: Robert A. Hatcher et al., "Menstrual Problems," *Contraceptive Technology 1990-1992* (New York: Irvington, 1990).

Osteoporosis and Diet

Osteoporosis, characterized by thinning of the bones and susceptibility to fracture, commonly affects elderly people in modern society and gets progressively worse with age. Conventional medicine has treated this disease with increased consumption of dairy food and other foods high in calcium and calcium supplements. Current research suggests that excessive animal protein, not lack of dietary calcium, is the primary cause of this degenerative ill.

• The Inuit (Eskimo) have the highest osteoporosis rates in the world. In a study of 217 children, 89 adults, and 107 elderly Inuit in Alaska, researchers found that they had lower bone mineral content, onset of bone loss at an earlier age, and development of bone thinning with a greater intensity than white Americans. The scientists attributed the greater degeneration to the acidic effects of the Inuits' high meat diet.

Sources: R. Mazess and W. Mather, "Bone Mineral Content of North Alaskan Eskimos,"*American Journal of Clinical Nutrition* 27:916-25, 1974.

• A Michigan State study found that by age 65, the average woman who ate meat had lost one-third of her skeletal structure. Meanwhile, vegetarian woman of comparable age had less than half the bone loss and were more active, less likely to break bones, maintained erect postures, and healed bones more quickly.

Source: F. Ellis et al., "Incidence of Osteoporosis in Vegetarians and Omnivores," *American Journal of Clinical Nutrition* 27:916, 1974.

• Researchers from Creighton University in Omaha, Nebraska, and Purdue University in West Lafayette, Indiana, reported that the calcium in kale is readily absorbed by the body and more efficiently than the calcium contained in milk. In studies of eleven women, the absorption of calcium from 300 mg. of kale averaged .409, while from a similar amount of milk calcium absorption averaged .321.

"We interpret our findings as evidence of good bioavailability for kale calcium and probably for the loss of low-oxalate vegetable greens as well," the researchers concluded. Other greens they listed included broccoli, turnip, mustard, and collard greens.

Source: Robert P. Heaney and Connie M. Weaver, "Calcium Absorption from Kale," *American Journal of Clinical Nutrition* 51: 656-57,1990.

• Drinking fluoridated water may increase the risk of hip fractures in older people. In a Utah study, women living in Brigham City which has added fluoride to its water supply since 1966 were 1.3 times more likely to suffer hip fractures than those living in two other communities that did not fluoridate their water.

Source: Christa Danielson et al., "Hip Fractures and Fluoridation in Utah's Elderly Population," *Journal of the American Medical Association* 268:746-48, 1992.

Breastfeeding and Cancer Prevention

• Breast-feeding can reduce the risk of certain cancers for both mother and child. Researchers from the National Institute of Child Health and Human Development in Bethesda, MD., found that infants breast-fed more than 6 months had a lower risk of developing cancer in childhood, especially lymphomas.

In this study, children who were formula-fed or breast-fed for less than six months had approximately twice the risk of getting some childhood cancers by age fifteen as those breast-fed for longer than 6 months. They also had five times the risk of getting lymphoma.

"Mother's milk contains substantial antimicrobial benefits for infants, increasing their resistance to many infections and possibly protecting them from many diseases, including lymphomas," researchers reported.

Source: "Breast-Feeding Linked to Decreased Cancer Risk for Mother, Child," *Journal of the National Cancer Institute* 80:1362-63, 1988.

• In a Chinese medical study, researchers found that the longer the mother nursed, the less at risk she was of breast cancer. Mimi Yu, Associate Professor of Preventive Medicine at the University of Southern California in Los Angeles, studied more than 500 Chinese women with breast cancer in Shanghai and 500 healthy women.

The women she studied on an average nursed their various children for a cumulative total of nine years, a common pattern in China. "We believe that long periods of nursing would have the same protective effect for American women," Yu reported.

Source: "Breast-Feeding Linked to Decreased Cancer Risk for Mother, Child," *Journal of the National Cancer Institute* 80:1362-63, 1988.

• An analysis of seventeen pesticides, toxins, and other chemical substances in the breast milk of vegetarian and nonvegetarian mothers found that except for polychlorinated biphenyls (which were about equal) "the highest vegetarian value was lower than the lowest value obtained in the [nonvegetarian] sample. . . . [T]he mean vegetarian levels were only one or two percent as high as the average levels in the United States."

Source: J. Hergenrather et al., "Pollutants in Breast Milk of Vegetarians," [Letter], *New England Journal of Medicine* 304:792, 1976.

Diet and Coronary Heart Disease

Although Americans are consuming less fat than previously, women on an average still consume 36 percent of their daily calories from fat, more than twice the recommended amount. Women who eat grain and vegetables and fish instead of land animals for protein have healthier hearts. Women who eat vegetables and fruits high in beta-carotene, Vitamin C, and other antioxidants can reduce their risk of heart attack by one-third. Dietary changes can also reduce obesity, which is associated with a threefold increase in coronary risk.

Source: Jane E. Brody, "The Leading Killer of Women: Heart Disease," *New York Times*, Nov. 10, 1993.

Menstruation and Heart Disease

Excess iron in the blood may be a primary cause of heart disease and double the risk of heart attacks in men. Finnish researchers theorized that iron in the bloodstream accounts for the higher rate of heart attacks in men than in young women, whose iron levels decline during menstruation.

About 50 percent of the dietary iron in the Finnish study came from animal food sources.

Source: "High Stored Iron Levels Are Associated with Excess Risk of Myocardial Infarction in Eastern Finnish Men," *Circulation* 86:803-11, 1992.

Stroke and Diet

Women who eat plenty of vegetables and fruits have a 54 percent lower rate of stroke than women with vitamin-poor diets, according to researchers at the American Heart Association's annual epidemiology meeting in Santa Fe.

Source: "Studies Tie Diets High in Vitamins to Reduced Stroke and Heart Ills," *Boston Globe*, March 19, 1993.

Breast Cancer and Primitive Society

American women are 100 times more at risk for breast cancer than their Stone Age sisters, scientists reported at the annual meeting of the American Association for the Advancement of Science. Currently, 1 in 9 women gets breast cancer. Stone Age practices such as early child-birth, breast-feeding, late menarche, lower estrogen levels, and healthier diet should reduce this rate to 1 in 900.

Source: *One Peaceful World Journal*, Spring 1993

Women's Health Resources

The Women's Health Seminar, a new weekend program at the Kushi Institute, focuses on common ailments, conditions, and issues women are facing today including PMS, cancer, breast disease, infertility, osteoporosis, menopause, candida, and vaginal infections. For information, please contact the Kushi Institute, Box 7, Becket, MA 01223 (413) 623-5741, fax (413) 623-8827.

The Women's Macrobiotic Society sponsors activities and events of interest to women. For information, please contact Gale Jack, coordinator, Box 172, Becket, MA 01223.

One Peaceful World is an international macrobiotic information network and friendship society with thousands of members around the world. Annual membership dues are $30 ($40 outside of North America) and benefits include a subscription to the *One Peaceful World Journal* (with new recovery cases in each issue), a free book from OPW Press, discounts on other books and study materials. For information, please contact One Peaceful World, Box 10, Becket, MA 01223 (413) 623-2322, fax (413) 623-6042.

Recommended Reading

Aveline: The Life and Dream of the Woman Behind Modern Macrobiotics by Aveline Kushi, $20.00. Aveline's enchanting autobiography.

Aveline Kushi's Complete Guide to Macrobiotic Cooking by Aveline Kushi, $15.99. The best general cookbook, including Aveline's charming drawings and poems.

Basic Home Remedies by Michio Kushi, $6.95. Guide to Special Drinks, Plasters, Compresses, and Other Applications including many special female applications.

Cancer-Free: 30 People Who Recovered from Cancer Naturally by Ann Fawcett, $20.00. Stories of ordinary people, who recovered from a wide variety of cancers.

Diet for Natural Beauty by Avleine Kushi with Wendy Esko and Maya Tiwari, $27.00. A natural anti-aging formula for skin and hair care.

Promenade Home: Macrobiotics and Women's Health by Gale and Alex Jack, $18.95. Gale's story about healing ovarian tumors and many other conditions and an introduction to macrobiotics and women's health.

Recovery from Cancer by Elaine Nussbaum, Avery Publishing Group, $9.95. The moving story of a mother who had inoperable uterine cancer and was told she had only a short time to live.

Rice Is Nice by Wendy Esko, $8.95. 108 Quick and Easy Brown Rice Recipes.

These and other books are available from One Peaceful World Press, Box 10, Becket, MA 01223. Make checks payble to OPW or send Visa/MC information. Please add $3.00 per order for postage in the U.S. and Canada. Elsewhere add 25% of the total for surface postage and 50% for airmail postage.

Contributors

Gladys Abeashie lives in Ghana.

Chris Akbar lives at the Kushi House in Brookline, Mass.

Lucy Burdo studied at the Kushi Institute and is now writing a cookbook in Putney, Vermont, where she lives.

Marlene Barrera lives in Plano, Texas, and directs a Spanish ministry program at a local church.

Martha Cottrell, M.D., served as medical director at the Fashion Institute of Technology in New York for many years. She is co-author with Michio Kushi of *AIDS, Macrobiotics, and Natural Immunity*.

Helen Farrell, M.D., lives in Canada and specializes in treating PMS and related conditions.

Edward Esko teaches at the Kushi Institute and internationally. He is the author of *Healing Planet Earth*.

Wendy Esko teaches at the Kushi Institute, is the author of *Rice Is Nice* and other cookbooks, and co-founder of *Ki Essentials*, a natural cosmetics company.

Dawn Gilmour lives in North Carolina. She teaches macrobiotic cooking throughout the United States and Europe.

Virginia Harper is a macrobiotic cook and teacher living in Franklin, Tennessee.

Yukio Horio works for a publishing company in Tokyo.

Alex Jack is director of One Peaceful World Press and co-author with Michio Kushi of *The Cancer-Prevention Diet*.

Gale Jack is director of the Women's Macrobiotic Society, a cooking teacher at the Kushi Institute, and author of *Promenade Home: Macrobiotics and Women's Health*.

Janet Karovitz resides in Montreal, Canada.

Michio Kushi is the leader of the macrobiotic community.

Kathleen Raeder lives in Aurora, Colorado.

Joan Young lives in North Brunswick, New Jersey.

Index